W9-AWZ-306

P
E
P

Sneezing Your Head Off?

How to Live with Your Allergic Nose

PETER B. BOGGS, M. D.

P
E
P

Sneezing Your Head Off?

Copyright © 1992, 1994 by Peter B. Boggs, M.D.

All rights reserved, including the right of
reproduction in whole or in part in any form.

ISBN 0-9642569-0-8

Manufactured in the United States of America

The ideas, procedures, and suggestions contained in this book are not
intended to replace the services of a trained health professional. All matters
regarding your health require medical supervision. You should consult your
physician before adopting the procedures in this book. Any applications of
the treatments set forth in this book are at the reader's discretion.

For Mary, Mary Elizabeth, and Doodle

ACKNOWLEDGMENTS

SO MANY PEOPLE have played a role in this book: My father, H. Whitney Boggs, Sr., M.D., who was the first physician and the first allergist in my life; my brother, H. Whitney Boggs, Jr., M. D., a colon and rectal surgeon who gave his support and brothership; my mother, Chastine Boggs, who was always my supporter; my first partner in the practice of medicine, Albert L. Stephens, Jr., M.D., who was such a good physician and friend.

Special appreciations go to "The Chief," John P. McGovern, M.D., founder of the McGovern Allergy Clinic in Houston, Texas, and under whom I trained, who provided an enormous clinical opportunity from which I learned, and to O. C. Thomas, M.D., who took me under his wing.

Each of us has a teacher or teachers somewhere in our past that "made the difference." Mine were Miss Elizabeth Mills, Mr. Leonard Oldham, and Mr. Leonard Opdyke. There are simply no words to express the gratitude I feel for these wonderful, caring people. Had they not been there, at that time. . . .

I am especially indebted to my writing mentor, thriller writer Harold King. Although busy with his own novel, not only did he give me encouragement, he spent many hours reading and advising on this text, and, in the process, he became a friend. Helping others is Hal's way, and I will forever be appreciative. Thanks also to Elaine King for reading the text, commenting, asking questions, and always offering words of encouragement.

Appreciations to my friend Edward J. O'Connell, M.D., for his editorial comments, willingness to write the foreword, and friendship over the years.

I want to thank all the patients over the years for their trust and their wanting to know.

Thanks to my office staff, who have helped in so many ways: Shirley, Millie, Vicki, Renee, Wanda, Janelle, Mona, Suzanne, Lynn, Virginia, and Dennis. And thanks to my partner, Willard F. Washburne, M.D., for our years in practice and for his friendship.

Thank you Henry Morrison, for being willing to take a chance. And to my editors, Toni Sciarra and Jennifer Trachtenberg, whose comments and editorial changes were thoughtful, helpful, and served to make this a better book. Appreciations to Jim Wilson for the artwork in this text.

To special friends, Dave and Becky White, thanks.

Most special appreciations to my family: my wife Mary and my daughters Mary Elizabeth and Doodle. Their love and support of me is as much a part of this book as the words I have placed on these pages.

CONTENTS

PART THREE
Conditions That Masquerade As Allergic Rhinitis

PART FOUR
Getting to Know *Your* Nose

PART FIVE
Taking Care of Your Nose

PART SIX
Complications of Rhinitis

FOREWORD

FIFTY MILLION PEOPLE suffer from nasal congestion, a runny nose, itchy eyes, or severe headaches. In most cases these symptoms indicate an allergic reaction. In fact, allergies and infections of the nose, sinuses, and ears are some of the most common ailments observed in medicine. Despite the prevalence of these problems there hasn't been a book that helps allergy sufferers find information on the diagnosis and treatment they need.

Until *Sneezing Your Head Off?* by Dr. Peter Boggs was written, most of the available information about allergies existed only in pamphlet form and was often too brief, inaccurate, or misleading. Now, Dr. Boggs has simplified a very complex subject and presents it to the reader in an organized fashion. Dr. Boggs is a well-trained board-certified allergist/immunologist of national respect who has a wealth of experience from years of practice and teaching. He remains on the cutting edge in this field and effectively conveys his expertise in this book.

Sneezing Your Head Off? discusses the anatomy and physiology of the nose, sinuses, ears, and upper respiratory system (complete with excellent anatomic diagrams), identifies and explains the various conditions affecting these areas, including symptoms of various allergies, and discusses and evaluates treatments. This book is intended to be supplemental to your physician's diagnosis and treatment, but is also designed to be a self-help volume for those wishing to obtain additional information and greater understanding of these problems.

As an allergist I found it interesting and exciting to learn from *Sneezing Your Head Off?* about rhinitis and related conditions. I am certain that this book will be widely accepted and fill a large void in patient information about these common maladies. This instructional volume will be the one that I recommend to my patients.

—Edward J. O'Connell, M.D., Professor of Pediatrics, Allergy/ Immunology, Mayo Medical School, Mayo Graduate School and Foundation, Rochester, Minnesota

HOW THIS BOOK CAN HELP YOU

THIS BOOK is about allergic noses and the conditions that masquerade as allergic noses. It's about sniffing and sneezing. It's about drippy noses, stopped-up noses, and itchy noses. It's about pollens, dusts, dogs, cats, and house mites. It's about allergy tests, skin-testing, and blood testing; antihistamines, decongestants, corticosteroid sprays, and cromolyn sodium; allergy desensitization shots and blood pressure pills. It's about bloody noses, infected sinuses, fluid in the ears, and losing your sense of smell. This book is about noses, all about noses, and the problems they cause.

And they cause a lot of problems:

- More than 1 *billion* people worldwide suffer because of their noses, some 50 *million* of those here in the United States.
- Nose problems make you feel miserable, they embarass you, keep you awake at night, give you headaches, and cause you to be unable to concentrate at work or at school.
- Nose problems send you to the doctor and they cause you to take medication(s), which sometimes makes you feel even worse.
- Nose problems are expensive. In the United States alone, nasal sufferers lose about $200 million in wages and spend almost $1 billion in health care delivery every year.
- Each year, in the United States alone, nasal sufferers lose some 5 million days from work and 3 million days from school.

Despite all of these nasal statistics, however, most people don't know one "hoot" about their noses.

This book will help you understand the following:

- How noses are made and how they work
- What it means to be allergic
- The various types of allergic nasal disorders
- How you become allergic, and to what types of agents you can become allergic
- All about indoor allergens: dust, mites, mold spores, dogs, and cats
- All about outdoor allergens: tree pollens, grass pollens, weed pollens, and outdoor molds
- What happens in your nose when an allergic reaction takes place
- All about early, late, dual, and delayed allergic reactions
- That what you thought was just one type of nasal problem could be two, three or even four different problems
- How to tell if you have hay fever and perennial allergic rhinitis
- Why your nose seems to be "twitchy," reacting to almost everything
- About nose conditions that masquerade as allergies and confuse both patients and physicians
- About allergy skin-tests and blood tests
- Why just vacuuming won't work to eradicate allergy causing house mites
- Why your "inside" cat should be outside
- The latest news about antihistamines, decongestants, and prescription antihistamine-decongestant combinations
- How to select over-the-counter nose medications
- The safest ways to take corticosteroid nasal sprays, cromolyn sodium spray, and a new medication called ipratropium bromide
- Who needs allergy shots and how they work
- Treatment cautions for nose patients with such special circumstances as pregnancy, breast feeding concerns, high

blood pressure, glaucoma, diabetes, heart problems, and urinary tract infections
- How to handle sinusitis
- What to do about ear infections and chronic fluid in the ears

This book is written for the millions of people who suffer from allergic and nonallergic nose symptoms. It is meant to be used in conjunction with your physician's treatment to help you better understand the type or types of nose problems you have, how they are diagnosed, the complications that they cause, and the treatment options available to you. I hope that it will help you become a more informed participant in the management of your chronic nasal symptoms so that you will miss fewer days of work or school, lose fewer nights' sleep, spend less money on health care, and generally enjoy an improved quality of life.

QUESTIONS, PLEASE

We all learn by asking questions. At the end of each chapter, you will find a section entitled "Questions and Answers." Here I will answer questions that patients commonly ask. I hope you will find these helpful and informative.

Speaking of questions, you might find the following to be of interest:

"Should I read this whole book?"
It is best to read this book from beginning to end, particularly if you have a nose problem but don't know whether or not you're allergic, or if you don't understand the types of nose problems you have.

"How do I use this book if I know what type of nose problem I have?"
While anyone with a nose problem should read chapter 1, "What Everyone Should Know About Noses," if your nose problem (s) already have been identified by a physician, then feel free to jump

to the sections that apply to your specific condition(s).

"My nose runs and I sneeze a lot, mainly in September and October? How should I use this book?"

If you have symptoms only during a single pollen season, be sure to read chapters 3 to 6. These chapters will help you understand what it means to be allergic as well as provide specific information about seasonal nasal allergy (hay fever) and the agents that cause it. Then read part 5, chapters 11 to 18, where you will learn about your treatment options.

"My nose is stopped up all year long. In fact, if I don't use a nose spray each night before I go to bed, the stuffiness awakens me periodically all night. What should I do?"

Turn to chapter 8: If It's Not an Allergy, What Is It? and read the section about "The Nose Drop Nose." Then call your doctor, tell him or her that you're "hooked" on nasal sprays, and ask him or her to help you get off of them. Nowdays, getting unhooked from nasal sprays is as easy as getting hooked, but you'll need your doctor's help. I've found that a combination of nasal decongestants, a short course of oral steroids, and the use of steroid nasal sprays quickly reverses the damage caused by abusing over-the-counter, nasal decongestant sprays.

"I have chronic allergic nasal symptoms, but I also have high blood pressure and hardening of the coronary arteries. I've been told that I can take only plain antihistamines for my symptoms. How can I use this book?"

Be sure to read chapters 11 and 12, which cover in detail the topic of antihistamines and decongestants. Of particular importance are the sections concerning side effects and cautions. In addition, chapters 15 to 17 explain the proper use of steroid nasal sprays, cromolyn sodium nasal spray, ipratropium bromide nasal spray, and additional medications you might be able to use. Look them over, then ask your doctor what he or she recommends.

"I am plagued by allergies all year long: ragweed pollen in the fall, tree and grass pollen in the spring, my dog who has slept

with me for 10 years, house mites, and my friend's cat all cause me misery. I take three different types of medication and still don't get relief. Help!"

Because you need to understand all about allergic noses, their causes, and how they are diagnosed and treated, you should read chapters 1 to 18. Concentrate especially on the sections describing cats and mites as allergens, and how to reduce your exposure to them inside the home. It is important that you understand the uses of prophylactic medications as well, so read chapters 16 and 17, which explain about steroid and cromoloyn sodium nasal sprays. Then, look over the other chapters and read whatever you and your doctor feel applies to you.

"My grandson has horrible nasal allergy and is taking several different medicines that I administer when he visits during the weekend. I just want to learn more about allergies. Will this book help me do that?"

Yes, it will. You can read about each of the agents to which your grandson is allergic and learn how to better avoid them. You also can understand more about the medications he takes: what they are, what they do, and what their possible side-effects are.

Now, on to part 1, which provides basic information about how noses work and how they become allergic.

PART ONE

Normal Noses

CHAPTER 1

WHAT EVERYONE SHOULD KNOW
ABOUT NOSES

This chapter explains what everyone with an allergic or "twitchy" nose should know about noses:

- The basic structure of your nose and the names of its anatomical parts
- How your nose prepares the air you breathe for safe entry into your lungs
- How your nose cleans and protects itself
- How swollen noses affect your sense of smell

Reading this section with a mirror nearby so you can look at your own nose might aid your understanding of the noses structure.

THE EXTERNAL NOSE

THE EXTERNAL NOSE—the part you see when you look in the mirror—comprises only a small percentage of the total nose. Most of your nose is inside your skull, between your eyes, below your brain and above your mouth (figure 1-1).

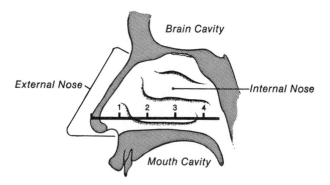

Figure 1-1: The Nose

This larger, internal part of your nose is appropriately called the **internal nose**. The space it occupies in your skull is called the **nasal cavity** (anatomists generally refer to spaces as "cavities").

External Landmarks

Your **external nose** begins at your forehead at the **ROOT** (figure 1-2) and extends along what is commonly called the bridge (or **DORSUM**) to its tip (known anatomically as the **APEX**). Then it curls under and seems to end just above your lip, with nostril openings for air on either side. The area between the **TIP** and where the nose meets the skin of the upper lip is called the **BASE** (figure 1-2). At the base of your nose are the **nares**, also known as the **nostrils**, the **alae** (meaning "wings"), which are walls surrounding the nostrils, and the column-like structure that separates your nostrils called the **columnella**.

Using a mirror, look carefully at your nostrils. Note that just where your skin changes into the pink lining of your nose, there are many hairs, called **vibrissae**. These prevent unwanted particles from entering your nose and, by extension, your lungs. These can become a nuisance if the tiny follicles associated with each become inflamed.

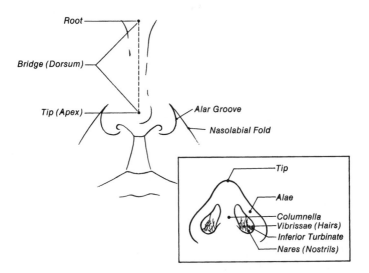

Figure 1-2: The External Nose

The grooves where the "wings" or alae that surround your nostrils join your cheeks are called the **alar grooves**. At the top of each groove and running toward the corner of your mouth is a fold of skin called the **nasolabial fold**. These folds become more prominent as we age.

Bones and Cartilages of the External Nose

Push on your nose near the **root**. It is firm because the **nasal bones** form this upper third of your nose (figure 1-3). This rigid upper third of your external nose is called the **bony bridge**.

Now push anywhere on your nose from just above the middle of the **bridge** to the **tip**. Flexible, right? This is because cartilage, not bone, forms the lower two-thirds of your nose. Cartilage is part of the framework upon and around which our body tissues exist, but cartilage is less dense and more flexible than bone. The **upper lateral cartilages** and the **lower lateral cartilages** form the main portion of the nose, with the support of several lesser cartilages known as the **accessory cartilages**. Together these form the **cartilagenous bridge**. If this lower two thirds of your external nose weren't flexible, think of how many times your nose would have been broken.

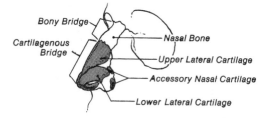

Figure 1-3: Bones and Cartilages of the External Nose

Note how the **lower lateral cartilages** curve to form the alae. It's this special wing-like shape of these lower cartilages, plus some fat and connecting tissue, that gives support to this outer wall of your nostrils, holding them open so that you can breathe effectively.

THE INTERNAL NOSE: THE NASAL CAVITY

The two-thirds of your nose that you don't see when you look in the mirror is a very intricately constructed cavity placed in your skull between your brain cavity above and your oral or mouth cavity below. It's larger than you might think: its upper boundary begins at the root of the nose and extends straight back 10 to 12 centimeters, or 4 to 5 inches.

The Nasal Septum

Your **nasal cavity** is divided vertically by a wall, **the nasal septum**, running roughly down the middle throughout the entire depth of the cavity. The septum is composed of bone and cartilage and is actually a conglomeration of some nine separate bones (figure 1-4).

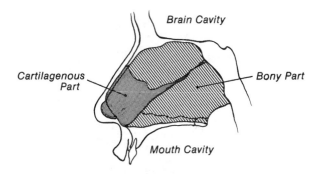

Figure 1-4: The Nasal Septum

Not everyone's septum is straight like a wall dividing two rooms. Some bend or curve slightly to the right or left side of the nasal cavity, deviations that normally cause no problems. If it curves too much, however, the septum is said to be deviated and can partially or completely block one side of the nose. Almost everyone has some deviation of their nasal septum, but only about 15 to 20 percent of the people in the United States have enough deviation to cause symptoms: one-sided nasal blockage or stuffiness, or increased postnasal drainage.

The Lateral or Side Walls of the Nasal Cavity

You can't see the right or left side walls of the nose well by just looking into your nostrils. Doctors have to use special instruments to see this part of your nose. The side walls of the nose (figure 1-5) are formed by the cheek bones. Three oblong extensions, called **conchae** or **turbinates**, arise from the side wall and form its most prominent landmarks. The smallest and highest placed conchae is the **superior turbinate**, next in size and location is the **middle turbinate**, and the largest and the one closest to the floor of the nose is the **inferior turbinate**.

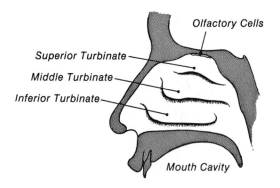

Figure 1-5: Side Wall of Nose

If you tilt your head slightly backwards and peek into your nostrils, you can see pink fingertip-like structures on the right and left side wall of your nose. These are the front tips of the inferior turbinate (figure 1-2). That's really about all you can see of these turbinates without using special instruments.

Each of your turbinates curves downward away from the side wall in such a manner as to create a space between itself and the side wall (look again at figure 1-5). These spaces are very important, as they control the flow of air into and through your nose and ensure close contact of air with the mucous membrane lining of the nose. Each space, or meatus (an anatomical term for space), is named for the turbinate causing its formation. Thus, the **superior meatus** lies under the superior turbinate, the **middle meatus** is located under the middle turbinate, and the **inferior meatus** is under the inferior turbinate. The largest and most important of the spaces is the middle meatus. It is the most important because of its size, because it does much of the work of the nose (see below), and because it is the space into which three major sinus cavities (frontal, maxillary, and ethmoid sinuses) drain. The other sinuses and the **nasolacrimal duct** drain into the other spaces (figure 1-6).

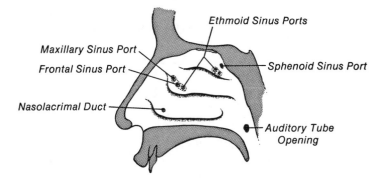

Figure 1-6: Drainage Ports of the Nose

The nasolacrimal duct is the tube through which your body removes excess tears from your eyes. Tears are constantly made by your tear glands, and those that aren't required to lubricate your eyes must be removed; otherwise, you'd look as if you were crying all the time. Your nasolacrimal duct works like this: Excess tears are drawn into a sac-like structure between the corner of your eye and the root of your nose. When you blink, the sac is compressed and the tears are squeezed out of the sac into the nasolacrimal duct. They drain into the nose in the front portion of the inferior meatus.

The maxillary sinuses ("sinus" is another anatomical name for a space or cavity), frontal sinuses, and part of the ethmoid sinuses drain into the nose through a long groove-like opening toward the front of the middle meatus. The remaining ethmoids drain into the the superior meatus. The sphenoid sinuses open into your nose via a groove-like opening just above the superior meatus.

This close relationship between your nose and sinuses makes it easy to see how your sinuses can become infected when your nose is infected, or how your nose can become infected when your sinuses are infected. Sinusitis, or infected sinuses, is discussed in chapter 19.

One other opening in the lateral wall of your nose that you should know about is the **auditory tube opening**. Through this opening your middle ear connects to your nose by a tube called the

eustachian tube. Note that the auditory tube opening is located just behind the inferior turbinate, where the nose opens into the pharynx. Given this location, it is easy to understand how the ears can become infected when the nose is infected. Infected ears and fluid in the ears are discussed in chapter 20.

The Mucous Membrane Lining of the Nose

The cells predominantly found in the lining of the nose are called **pseudostratified ciliated columnar epithelial cells.** These cells are tall, like columns, and have hair-like projections called cilia extending from their tops (figure 1-7). These ciliated cells are covered by a blanket of mucus produced by various glands and cells within the lining membrane. This mucus blanket has two layers: an upper, sticky, chunky layer called the **gel** (for *gel*atinous) layer and a lower, thin, watery layer called the **sol** (for *sol*ution), which is just thick enough to cover the cilia projecting upward from the lining cells. How this layer traps particles and how these trapped particles are removed from the nose is discussed below under "What Your Nose Does for You."

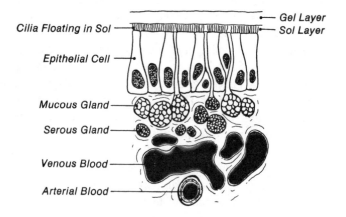

Cilia Floating in Sol — Gel Layer / Sol Layer
Epithelial Cell
Mucous Gland
Serous Gland
Venous Blood
Arterial Blood

Figure 1-7: Mucous Membrane of Nose

The lining membrane of your nose contains a variety of other cells that protect you from noxious agents and infection. They also can participate in allergic reactions. These will be discussed later under the specific types of rhinitis in which they play a major role. Underneath the lining cells is a rich supply of nerve tissue, lymphatics, and blood vessels. This supply is especially abundant over the three turbinates. This portion of the nasal membrane is "erectile"; it actually functions very similarly to penile tissue in its ability to fill and empty with blood and to distend when engorged with blood. This response is most prominent in that portion of the lining membrane covering the turbinates, and is most pronounced over the inferior turbinate.

WHAT YOUR NOSE DOES FOR YOU

Your nose does much more than let you breathe with your mouth closed and function as your organ of smell. It warms and humidifies the air you breathe; it filters, entraps, and eliminates unwanted particles and gases; it kills unwelcome bacteria and viruses; it acts as a resonating chamber when you speak; and it reabsorbs water from the air you expire. It also prepares the air you breathe for entry into your lungs. Let's learn a little more about each of these important functions of the nose.

Sense of Smell

The cells of smell in the lining of the nose, the **olfactory cells**, are located high in the nasal cavity in the area above the superior turbinate (look back at figure 1-5). Necessary for a normal sense of smell is the regular flow of air across these olfactory cells. This, of course, requires a normally open nose. We've all experienced a reduction or inability to smell when our noses stop up from a cold or a bad allergic reaction. In addition, when our sense of smell is reduced, so is our sense of taste. Our enjoyment of the taste of food is the result of a simultaneous stimulation of the olfactory cells in our noses and the taste buds in our mouths. When the odors do not reach the olfactory cells because of a stopped-up nose, our food becomes less enjoyable.

Conduction of Air

Under normal conditions, when you breathe through your nose, air enters the nose through the **nostrils** and then follows one of three general courses through the nose (figure 1-8).

The majority of the air you inhale is directed through the large, slitlike middle meatus passageway lying between the middle turbinate and the lateral wall of the nasal cavity, and thus over the top of the inferior turbinate.

About 10 percent of the air you breathe is directed to the ceiling or vaulted area of the nose. It then travels toward the back of the nose, passing across a special area of the lining of the hose, the **organ of smell**, in its course. The organ of smell is the structure with which we sense odors in the air we breathe. The remainder of inspired air traverses the nose either through the inferior meatus passageway along the **floor** of the nose or along the septum.

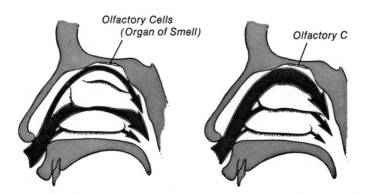

Figure 1-8: Normal Air Flow and Sniffing

All the air that goes through the normal nose passes through these narrow, slit-like passageways, usually only 1 to 3 millimeters wide. This means that the air is in very close contact with the mucous membrane lining of the nose throughout its journey through the nose.

Because of the curves and grooves formed by the turbinates, septum, and conchae, normal air flows through the slit-like nasal passageways (figure 1-8) in either a very smooth, or a tumbling, stumbling manner. When the flow is smooth it is called laminar flow. Air flows through the vault of the nose and over the organ of smell area in a laminar manner. The smooth, even flow provides optimal sensing of the air you inspire by your organ of smell. In contrast, when the flow is tumbling, it is called turbulent. Over the lower portions of the nose, air flow is turbulent. This uneven, tumbling flow hurls inspired particles about like a wind storm and facilitates their entrapment in the sticky mucus surface of the lining membrane of the nose, keeping them from passing into your lungs.

You've probably sniffed food, flowers, or a good wine many times. Ever wonder why the act of sniffing seems to sharpen your sense of smell? The process of sniffing actually changes the pattern of air flow through your nose. During sniffing, more air is directed high into your nose, across the area where it is sampled by your olfactory cells. The better the sample, the better your ability to sense odors.

Some 10,000 liters of air pass through the normal adult nose every 24 hours. In spite of this high volume of air passing through such tiny passageways, normal nose breathing takes place unnoticed and without conscious effort.

Warming and Humidification

Your nose prepares air for entry into your lower airways and lungs by warming and humidifying it. The nose is an ideal air conditioning system. Even extremely cold and dry air will be warmed almost to body temperature and completely humidified in the few milliseconds it takes for air to traverse your nose and pass through the voice box into the lungs. Your nose does this every time you take a breath, 24 hours each day. That is one heck of an air conditioning system.

Making this process possible are the numerous mucus secreting glands and cells of the lining of your nose and sinuses and the fluids they produce. Intimate contact between the air and this fluid layer permits transfer of water from the nasal mucus into the dry inspired air.

Filtration

Your nose is also a remarkable filter. Particulate matter such as dust, mold spores, pollens, bacteria, viruses, and even some gases are completely removed by the nose from the air before it enters the lungs. Almost nothing as large as a pine pollen grain (much smaller than a grain of salt) ever makes it through the nose. This is an imperfect system, however, and some very tiny particles will find their way into the lower airways, which may give rise to airway irritation, infection, or asthma.

Certain pollutant gases such as sulphur dioxide and ozone, as well as formaldehyde, are filtered by the nose. They are actually absorbed by the gel layer of the mucus lining of the nose, and then swept clear of the nose by the efforts of the mucociliary clearance mechanism described below.

Mucociliary Clearance

Each of your lining cells has about 25 cilia that exist in a state of constant, rhythmic, sweeping motion (some 250 times per minute). The motion of the cilia is highly coordinated, and their sweeping action moves the chunks of gel with its trapped particles in a wave-like flow toward either the back or the front of your nose. Particles entrapped in the rear two-thirds of the nose are swept to the back of your nose and swallowed. Particles entrapped in the front part of the nose, before reaching the turbinates, are swept to your nostrils where they dry, become encrusted and are generally removed by nose blowing.

Resonation of our Voices

The nasal cavity enriches and amplifies sound as we talk, giving a resonance to our voice that we would not otherwise have. I'm sure you've experienced a loss of quality of your voice when your nose was stopped-up by a cold, thus dampening the resonating ability of your nose.

Bacterial and Viral Killing

Foreign agents such as bacteria or viruses invading the nose run into what I call the Navy SEALS of the nose: the enzymes, cells, and antibodies of the mucosa, which are designed to immobilize and kill these invading terrorists.

THE NASAL CYCLE

The erectile quality of the membranes overlaying the turbinates brings us to something you may have noticed and been puzzled by: how one side of your nose can be stuffy while the other side is clear.

Believe it or not, every day, 24 hours a day, the membranes on one side of your nose will engorge with blood while those on the opposite side of your nose empty. This phenomenon is so regular, occurring every 1 to 4 hours (it varies from one person to another) that it is called the **nasal cycle.**

Why our noses work this way is not known, but it probably has something to do with keeping the lining cells of the nose healthy so they can function properly. It's akin to a work-rest cycle. This nasal cycle is noticeable only when something "twitches" your nose-like a cold, an allergy, or an addiction to nasal sprays-and exaggerates or prolongs the cycle.

NOSE SYMPTOMS

Almost any of what allergists call triggering or "twitching" agents, be it infection, allergy, or irritant, çan cause any of the symptoms listed below:

Stuffy or stopped-up nose	Runny nose/sniffing
Sneezing	Itching
Burning	Increased drainage of
Bleeding	mucus down the back
Decreased or complete loss	of your throat
of sense of smell	Pain

These symptom occur because something has interfered with one or more of the normal functions of the nose. For example:

When this happens	*Your nose gets*
Air passageways narrow	Stuffy, blocked-up
Mucous glands increase flow	Runny, heavy drainage
Mucous glands decrease flow	Dry, painful, bloody
Mucociliary clearance fails	Dry, crusted, infected
Bacterial/viral killing fails	Infected
Air doesn't pass over your organ of smell	Reduced or loss of smell
Lining membrane is cut	Bleeding
Special nerve cells are stimulated	Itching, sneezing, pain

TEN TRUTHS THAT EVERYONE SHOULD KNOW ABOUT NOSE SYMPTOMS

1. There are many agents that can trigger or twitch your nose: dust, pollen, dogs, cats, cold air, infections, smoke, bright lights, etc. These will be discussed in detail in chapters 5 to 8.

2. Most people with twitchy noses have more than one twitching agent.
3. More than one twitcher may stimulate your nose at any one time, and they frequently do.
4. You may not be aware of all the agents responsible for your symptoms, although you'll be much more aware after reading this book.
5. Twitchy noses run, drip, sniff, sneeze, drain, stuff-up, stop-up, itch, burn, bleed, and occasionally hurt, and do so in various combinations.
6. The type of symptom most annoying to you may change from day to day, or even hour to hour: runny now, sneezing in 2 hours, stopped-up tonight, itchy in the morning.
7. What twitches you doesn't necessarily twitch someone else.
8. Even if it does, your symptoms may differ from someone else's symptoms.
9. Even if your symptoms are similar to someone else's, you will each differ in your degree of discomfort.
10. The specific medication(s) that help your twitchy nose may or may not help mine.

In the next chapter, we'll talk about **allergic noses**: what it really means to have an allergic nose, the types of allergic noses, and the agents to which we can become allergic.

QUESTIONS AND ANSWERS

1. My sense of smell is not as good as it used to be. My doctor says it's because I have nasal polyps. How do they interfere with my sense of smell?

Nasal polyps commonly arise from an area high in the roof or vault of your nose. They are balloon-like swellings of the lining of your nose and crowd the tissue that surrounds them. If they occur near your olfactory area, they can block the flow of air through that part of your nose so that odors cannot be sensed.

If this happens, your sense of smell will be reduced or obscured completely

2. My nose seems to run all the time. Where does all that fluid come from?

The nose is a great manufacturer of fluid. It does this through two different types of cells and some special glands. In fact, about a quart of nasal fluid drains unnoticed down the back of your throat every 24 hours. This is normal, so your brain thinks nothing of it. Only when this fluid increases significantly, as in allergic reactions, infections, or responses to irritants, does your brain take notice and alert you to the drainage.

3. If I go to the movies in the afternoon and it is still bright outside when I come out, I sneeze and sneeze and my nose runs. Am I allergic to sunlight?

In brief, the problem with sunlight that you are experiencing is actually a nerve reflex that involves the eyes and the nose. It works like the reflex that causes your leg to jump when the doctor strikes your knee tendon with a rubber hammer: a stimulus is applied (hammer hitting tendon) and a response, directed by your nervous system, follows (leg jumps). In your case the stimulus is sunlight striking the back of your eye, and the response is the glands of your nose rapidly making fluid and your sneezing mechanism being activated. Any bright light can do this.

4. If I have a cold and blow my nose, can I blow germs into my sinus cavities or ears?

You can, and that is one way that you can contract sinus and ear infections. It is better to gently sniff the mucus back into your throat and expel it than to blow your nose.

PART TWO

Allergic Noses

CHAPTER 2

WHAT ARE ALLERGIC NOSES?

ALLERGIC RHINITIS is the most common of all allergic disorders. *Rhinitis* is the general medical term for disorders of the nose in which an inflammation of the lining of the nose occurs and symptoms such as runny nose, sneezing, congestion, and drainage result. *Allergic Rhinitis* refers to the three types of nasal inflammatory disorders caused by allergic reactions: Seasonal Allergic Rhinitis, Perennial Allergic Rhinitis, and Occupational Allergic Rhinitis.

It is estimated that at any given time 20 percent of the US. population suffers from allergic rhinitis. That is the equivalent of the total population of the western one-third of the United States.

Each year allergic rhinitis results in 28 million days of restricted activity, 6 million days of bed rest, and 3 million days lost from school. In addition, each year five million days are lost from work, $200 million are lost in wages, and $500 million are spent on health care, all because of allergic rhinitis.

Allergic rhinitis generally begins before twenty years of age, with the greatest rate of onset being between twelve and fifteen years of age. However, we are vulnerable at any age, and allergists will occasionally see someone over eighty years old experiencing their first episode of hay fever.

The long term outlook for patients with allergic rhinitis varies. Usually, once symptoms develop, they gradually worsen. Although some symptoms will improve with time, most will not and their victims will suffer for many years. It is wrong to advise anyone that he or she is likely to "outgrow" allergic rhinitis in just a few years. This kind of advice is especially erroneous when applied to children. They may grow out of it, but the odds are against them.

Just how allergy specialists arrive at a diagnosis of the type(s) of nasal problems you have is discussed in detail in chapter 9.

THE THREE TYPES OF ALLERGIC RHINITIS

1. Hay Fever or Seasonal Allergic Rhinitis

This form of nasal allergy is the result of becoming allergic to the pollen(s) present during a particular pollen season, and thus symptoms occur only during that season. The patient is symptom free the remainder of the year. The term hay fever is a misnomer for seasonal allergic rhinitis, since most seasonal allergic rhinitis is neither caused by hay nor associated with fever.

Characteristic symptoms include nasal congestion; watery, runny nose; sneezing spells; and itching of the nose, throat, roof of the mouth, and deep inside the ears. Sneezing, sometimes in attacks of ten or more sneezes at a time, are not uncommon. Additionally, many patients experience a concomitant allergic reaction of the eyes manifested as itchy, watery, red eyes in which the whites of the eyes and the eyelids can swell.

The most common causes of hay fever are shown in table 2-1.

Seasonal Allergic Rhinitis Example #1.

Jane is thirty-five years old and has had fall hay fever for fifteen years. During the first week of September she begins to have an intermittent runny nose, occasional nasal itching, and some sneezing. Over the next two weeks this progresses to a twenty-four-hour-a-day problem that persists through mid-October. During most of this time she generally feels miserable and is not as attentive at work or at home as she wants to be. The over-the-counter medications that she takes either make her sleepy or give her stomach cramps. Diagnosis: seasonal allergic rhinitis, fall weed pollens, ragweed.

TABLE 2-1
The Causes of Hay Fever

Type	Cause
Fall hay fever	Weed pollens
Spring hay fever	
Early spring	Tree pollens
Late spring	Grass pollens
Mid winter hay fever	Mountain cedar (south central Texas)
Early spring through onset of winter	Mold spores

Seasonal Allergic Rhinitis Example #2.

William is ten years old. Last spring he had some trouble with what his parents thought was a cold. It happened again in mid-March this year, except it was worse: terrible sneezing spells; red, itchy, and watery eyes; and an almost constantly running nose. Allergy testing showed him to be reactive to elm and oak pollen, both typical early spring pollens in his area. Diagnosis: seasonal allergic rhinitis, early spring pollens, elm and oak.

Seasonal Allergic Rhinitis Example #3.

Sgt. JCD/USAF is thirty years old and has been stationed at Lackland AFB, San Antonio, Texas, for the last three years. A native of Rhode Island, he'd never had an allergy problem until this past January when he began having sneezing spells and itchy eyes anytime he was outside longer than about 20 minutes, especially on windy days. At first, he thought there was something wrong with his contact lenses, but on consultation with his physician he discovered that he'd become allergic to mountain cedar, a tree peculiar to that part of the country and a common cause of mid-winter hay fever in South-Central Texas. Diagnosis: seasonal allergic rhinitis, mid-winter pollen, mountain cedar.

2. Perennial Allergic Rhinitis

This form of nasal allergy is caused by becoming allergic either to a single agent to which one is exposed on a year-around basis or to multiple agents whose collective exposure results in perennial, or year-around, symptoms. The symptoms of perennial allergic rhinitis are similar to those of seasonal allergic rhinitis, except that they persist throughout the year and tend not to be as explosive.

Both seasonal and nonseasonal allergens contribute to the symptoms of perennial allergic rhinitis. Table 2-2 lists the more common causes.

TABLE 2-2
The Causes of Perennial Allergic Rhinitis

Environmental allergens
    House dust
    House dust mites
    Mold spores
    Dogs, cats, feather pillows
Seasonal allergens
    Tree pollens
    Grass pollens
    Weed pollens
Animals
    Dogs
    Cats
    Feather pillows
Occupational agents
Foods

Most textbooks list the primary causes of perennial allergic rhinitis to be the environmental or household allergens: dust, mites, mold spores, animals. These are substances to which we are exposed year-around. In reality, however, most people who suffer with allergic rhinitis all year are not only reactive to one or more of these agents, but also are allergic to multiple pollens as well. It is this collective assault of multiple agents on an allergic nose that results in the presence of symptoms all year round.

Also assaulting the nose and causing nasal symptoms are a group of agents that allergists refer to as non-allergic irritants. They cause symptoms by their *irritant quality* rather than by their ability to stimulate allergic reactions, and they can cause symptoms in almost anyone who is sufficiently exposed. The common nonallergic irritants are discussed in detail in chapter 5: cigarette smoke, aerosol sprays, inert particles in the air, winds, cold air, bright lights, scented cosmetics, an almost limitless variety of chemicals, and more.

Chronic Rhinitis Example #1.

Anne is twenty-eight years old and never had any trouble with her nose until six months ago. She first noticed some stuffiness of the nose at night. Then it progressed to daily symptoms, alternating between congestion, sneezing, and runny nose and intermittent itching of the nose and eyes. A detailed allergy history revealed that a year ago she had been given a Siamese cat, Ginger, whom she kept inside and who slept on her bed each night and much of the day while Anne worked. She admitted with some reluctance that petting the cat would sometimes make her nose and eyes run and cause her to sneeze, "but, never this bad!" The cat was the only agent definitely suggested by her history as a cause of symptoms.

Allergy skin tests confirmed that her only positive reaction was to cats. Ginger became an outside cat, and Anne's symptoms completely cleared over the course of about three months. Diagnosis: perennial allergic rhinitis, cat.

Chronic Rhinitis Example #2.

Paul is twenty-six years old and has had an "allergic nose" since he was twelve years old. Prior to last year his symptoms occurred only in the spring, from March through May. However, since last March his symptoms have been continuous. No medicine helped, so he consulted an allergist. A detailed history strongly suggested that house dust, the family dog, ragweed pollen, elm pollen, and grass pollen *all* triggered his symptoms. Additionally, nonallergic irritant triggers of symptoms included cigarette smoke and strong perfumes.

Allergy skin testing confirmed Paul's history and further pinpointed the problem with house dust to be the house dust mite. Paul's allergy problems had increased over time. He no longer just had seasonal allergic rhinitis but chronic allergic rhinitis. He was placed on a treatment program encompassing avoidance, symptomatic medication, and allergy desensitization injections. Diagnosis: perennial allergic rhinitis, environmentals and pollens.

3. Occupational Allergic Rhinitis

Occasionally, agents to which workers are exposed will cause allergic nasal symptoms. The symptoms are the same as those of seasonal or chronic allergic rhinitis but the causative agents are those unique to the workplace. In this form of allergic rhinitis, as in the other forms, symptoms tend to parallel the exposure of the allergic workers: Intermittent, occasional exposure produces intermittent, occasional symptoms. Daily exposure results in chronic daily symptoms.

Occupational allergic rhinitis will be covered in more detail in chapter 7.

Occupational Allergic Rhinitis Example #1.

Vicki is a twenty-five-year-old laboratory technologist who has worked in the animal lab at a university medical center for just over two years. She has been bothered with seasonal allergic rhinitis since childhood, but in the last three months she has begun to experience episodic paroxysms of runny nose, sneezing, and itchy, red eyes whenever she goes into the rat room. Yesterday afternoon, the janitor began sweeping the room while she was working in it and, in addition to her nasal symptoms, she began to cough and wheeze slightly. On consultation with an allergist, Vicki learned that she had become allergic to the proteins in rat urine, which can dry and get into the air in places like animal laboratories, especially during the cleaning of cages and the sweeping of floors. Furthermore, her symptoms had become too severe to permit continued exposure. Fortunately she was able to transfer to another research project that did not involve contact with rats or their urinary proteins. Diagnosis: occupational allergic rhinitis, rat urine.

QUESTIONS AND ANSWERS

1. If I move from one area of the country to another, how long will it take me to become allergic to the pollens in the new area?

General wisdom suggests that it takes two to three seasons of exposure for you to become allergic to the agents in the new area that were not present in your former area. Of course, if there are allergens common to both areas, as there frequently are, you may continue to have allergic symptoms as before, only, perhaps, at slightly different times of the year.

2. Is it true that people outgrow nasal allergies?

No, it isn't. In fact, there is data to suggest that although a small percentage of people get better, a larger percentage worsen. The most likely explanation for the myth about outgrowing nasal allergies is that the symptoms that were diagnosed as "allergy" and subsequently "outgrown" were not actually caused by an allergy but by nonallergic factors such as irritants or infection.

3. My son's nose bleeds frequently. His pediatrician says that this is common in allergic children. Is it really common, and how do those things he's allergic to make his nose bleed?

Bleeding from the nose is common in children with allergic rhinitis, either seasonal or chronic. It generally happens only occasionally and is almost always mild and readily stopped.

The agents to which your son is allergic don't actually cause the bleeding, they just trigger an allergic reaction that swells the nasal membrane, making it vulnerable to injury. Additionally, the lining of the nose is only a few cells thick near the openings of the nose and is easily cut. As mucus and trapped particles are swept toward the front of the nose, they dry and form crusts. When a child wipes or rubs a drippy or itchy nose, these dried, encrusted particles are scraped across the nasal mucous membrane, cutting it and making it bleed.

4. What is "Rose Fever"?

This is a term that has been used to describe late spring seasonal allergic rhinitis. Its name derives from the fact that roses are in bloom at that time. However, the allergic symptoms are not due to rose pollen but to the pollen of the trees and grasses that are pollenating at the same time.

CHAPTER 3

HOW DID YOU BECOME ALLERGIC?

SEVERAL FACTORS DETERMINE whether or not you will develop allergic rhinitis. These are listed in table 3-1:

TABLE 3-1
Factors Influencing the Development of Allergic Rhinitis

Genetics	Age
Exposure	Race
Geographic location	Sex
Pollution	Infection

Genetic Factors

In order for you to develop allergic rhinitis, you must have inherited the ability to form allergic antibodies, called IgE antibodies, to things like pollen, mites, animals, etc. This ability runs in families, but the exact manner of its transmission from generation to generation has been difficult to define. Recent work suggests that a small fraction of chromosome number six carries this ability.

What is clear about the inheritance of allergic illness is that one's chances of developing allergic rhinitis are increased when one parent suffers from it and further increased when both parents are afflicted. Only a small percentage of people born into families in which neither parent has allergic rhinitis will ever develop allergic rhinitis.

Exposure

One thing is for certain about allergic rhinitis: you must be exposed to the things to which you have the inherited ability to make IgE antibodies, or you cannot become allergic.

INHERITANCE + EXPOSURE = ALLERGY

Geographic Location

The effects of geographic location are largely those of exposure. If you change geography-local, regional, national, or international-your exposure may be altered for either better or worse.

Pollution

Pollutants in the outdoor or indoor air mainly function as irritants, stimulating nerve endings in already-irritated allergic noses and causing symptom-producing reflexes to occur. To date there is no evidence that natural exposure to outdoor pollutants plays a causative role in the development of allergic rhinitis.

Such is not true for indoor pollutants, however, specifically cigarette smoke and the fumes of natural gas. Maternal cigarette smoking has been shown to increase the likelihood of developing allergic respiratory disease in nonsmoking children. Chronic exposure to maternal cigarette smoking and natural gas fumes have been associated with increased upper and lower respiratory infections in children. (In these studies mothers were the primary caretakers of the children; thus, their smoking affected the children adversely. If the situation were reversed and the father was the primary caretaker at home, his smoking would have an adverse effect on the children.

Age

It is estimated that 80 percent of the people who suffer from allergic rhinitis have their first symptoms prior to twenty years of age, with many at less than ten years of age. Allergic rhinitis tends to begin early in life, gradually worsen over many years, then decline in old age. Its decline during old age is likely due to a decline in the ability of our immune systems to mount allergic responses. Spontaneous remission of symptoms sometimes occurs in early to mid-life, but only in 15 to 25 percent of patients with seasonal allergic rhinitis. Sufferers of perennial allergic rhinitis are much less likely to undergo spontaneous remission.

Nationality

The incidence of various allergic disorders does vary between countries, but the factors responsible for this have not yet been defined. Table 3-2 provides examples of the considerable variations between countries:

TABLE 3-2
Incidence of Allergic Rhinitis by Country

Country	Incidence
Australia-New Zealand	7%
Great Britain	8%
Switzerland	9%
USA	8-19%
Venezuela	19%

Sex

During childhood, about twice as many boys as girls suffer from allergic rhinitis. During late childhood and adolescence this sexual difference equalizes. During the midlife years, more men are affected than women, but this difference disappears as people pass into their 50s. The reasons for these sexual differences are not known.

Infection

The ubiquitous nature of upper respiratory infections precludes any definitive statement about their role in the causation of allergic rhinitis. But the fact that the spring and fall pollen seasons coincide with a time of increased viral upper respiratory illnesses, and the fact that infections can alter immune responses (increasing certain ones and decreasing others) invites further research into the relationship of infectious illnesses and the development of allergic illnesses.

HOW ALLERGIES HAPPEN

If you have the inherited ability to form IgE to some allergic substance and you are exposed sufficiently to that substance, you will then form IgE antibodies against that substance. Once these IgE antibodies are formed, they attach themselves to certain cells in the lining of your nose—mast cells and basophil cells—and await re-exposure to the substance responsible for their generation. When re-exposure occurs, the IgE antibodies bind with the substance. This binding initiates a sequence of events that culminate in the release of chemicals from the interior of the cell and from the cell wall into the nasal lining. These chemicals, called chemical mediators, cause small blood vessels to dilate, fill with blood, and leak fluid into the nasal tissue. Swelling of the lining of the nose results. Other mediators stimulate nasal nerves and mucus-producing cells. Still other mediators attract into the nasal tissue cells of inflammation, and these then contribute their own set of mediators to produce an ongoing inflammatory reaction. All of this creates what we call symptoms: nasal congestion, runny nose, drainage, sneezing, itching, and a twitchy nose.

Let's look at each of the components in this sequence in a little more detail.

The Allergy Antibody: IgE

Humans can produce five separate and distinct classes of antibodies. IgE antibodies, which react with the pollens, dusts, dogs, etc. to which we become allergic, are similar to other antibodies in that they are composed of two heavy and two light protein chains connected to one another by chemical bonds. IgE is unique among antibodies, however, in its ability to bind firmly and for a prolonged period of time to two types of cells found in the lining membrane of the nose, mast cells and basophil cells. Without this ability, IgE would cause little or no trouble and you would not have an allergic nose. The IgE antibody is able to attach to these cells because of a special structure called a binding site on one end of its heavy chains. The other end of the IgE molecule also has binding sites that bind to the allergen that triggered its development: pollen, mold, cat protein, etc. This process of allergen binding is highly specific. For example, IgE made to react with ragweed will not react with oak pollen or cat protein but only with ragweed. Your body makes IgE antibodies specifically for each agent to which your nose becomes allergic.

The Mast Cells and Basophil Cells

The mast cells are located deep in the lining membrane of the nose, generally near blood vessels and mucus-producing cells. The basophils are located primarily near the surface of the nasal lining. They are the first cells encountered by entering pollens and other allergens—and the first that are triggered to respond during an attack of allergic rhinitis. Each type of cell is able to produce a wide variety of chemical mediators for release during an allergic reaction (table 3-3). Some of these mediators, called preformed mediators, exist already formed in the cells, while others, the newly formed mediators, are formed only after an allergic reaction is triggered.

TABLE 3-3
Chemical Mediators of Mast Cells and Basophil Cells

Preformed Mediators:

Histamine	Eosinophil chemotactic factor
Chymase	Neutrophil chemotactic factor
Tryptase	Heparin
Acid hydrolaxes	

Newly Formed Mediators:

Leukotrienes	Prostaglandins
Thromboxanes	

The Binding of IgE To Mast Cells and Basophils

Just as IgE has a binding site, the mast cells and basophil cells have a receiving site, or receptor, for the IgE binding site. Although this receptor will accept only IgE molecules, it will accept *any* type of IgE molecule. So, attached to any single mast cell or basophil cell can be a variety of different IgE antibodies: some made against ragweed, some against Johnson grass pollen, another against oak pollen, etc. Thousands of IgE molecules bind to each of these cells.

Being "Sensitized"

At the very instant that two or more agent-specific IgE antibodies attach closely to one another on the surface of a mast cell or basophil cell, you are sensitized to that agent. That means that the next time your nose is exposed to the agent, your newly created, agent-specific IgE antibodies will bind with it and your mast cells and basophils will react to it in such a manner that you will develop allergic symptoms.

The Chemical Mediators of Allergic Rhinitis

Table 3-3 above listed all of the mediators known to be released from mast cells and basophils during an allergic reaction. Table 3-4 lists those that have been shown to play a role in allergic rhinitis as well as the symptoms that they produce.

TABLE 3-4
Chemical Mediators Causing Symptoms of Allergic Rhinitis

Mediator	Symptoms Produced
Histamine	Stuffy nose, runny nose, sneezing, itchy nose, itchy throat, itchy palate, itchy ears
Prostaglandin D2	Inflammation of nose
Leukotrienes	Runny nose, stuffy nose, inflammation

Each of these mediators exerts its effect by interacting with a receptor on the surface of a specific cell in the nasal tissue. Histamine, for example, binds to one of two types of receptors, called H 1 and H2 receptors. Tissue that doesn't contain either of these receptors cannot be acted upon by histamine. It is mainly through the H1 receptor that histamine stimulates tissues in your nose and causes allergic symptoms. Antihistamines and other medications used to treat allergic symptoms act by blocking the receptors through which the chemical mediators work. Thus, antihistamines work mainly by blocking the interaction of histamine with the H1 receptor. This process will be discussed in more detail in chapter 11.

QUESTIONS AND ANSWERS

1. My daughter developed allergic rhinitis when she was nine years old. She's eleven years old now and it seems to be getting worse. A colleague at work told me that her allergy would probably develop into asthma. Is that true?

In general, 30 percent of patients with allergic rhinitis develop asthma. Asthma is a disorder in which episodes of narrowing of the bronchial tubes, swelling of the lining of these tubes, and increased mucus production in the lungs occurs. This causes coughing, wheezing, and shortness of breath. Since 70 percent of patients with allergic rhinitis will not develop asthma, your daughter has a better chance of not developing asthma than she does in developing asthma. Her chances for developing asthma increase if there is someone else in the family with asthma.

2. If you develop both allergic rhinitis and asthma, which usually begins first?

While asthma usually is diagnosed earlier in life than allergic rhinitis, this is only because its symptoms are much more noticeable from the start than those of allergic rhinitis. The results of studies exploring this question tend to show allergic rhinitis beginning first. About one-third of the studies show the two disorders beginning at the same time.

3. Should I "take my sinuses to Arizona"?

Only for a vacation, not as a treatment for your pollen allergies. Pollens abound in Arizona, although they are from different sources compared to those of, say, New Jersey. If you think I'm kidding, just count the specialists in allergy and immunology in the yellow pages of the Phoenix and Scottsdale telephone directories. You can change your geography, but you can't change your genes. If you want to plan a vacation around the pollens that trigger your allergy symptoms, read chapter 5 and discuss your situation with your regular physician or allergist.

4. I've heard that a child born in the spring is more likely to become allergic later in life than one born in the winter. Is that true?

There is information to suggest that the risk of developing hay fever later in life is doubled in children who are born during grass pollen season. These findings need to be further researched in different geographic areas, for different pollen seasons, and by additional investigators before they can be accepted.

5. Both my husband and I are allergic and I'm pregnant. What are the chances that our child will be allergic?

If both of you are allergic, your child's chances of becoming allergic are between 50 and 75 percent. If just one of you is allergic, your child's chances are more like 25 to 50 percent. There is a small chance, about 10 percent, of your child being allergic even if neither of you have allergic symptoms. It is important to note that your child possesses a mixture of genes from you and your husband. How these combine will determine if and to what your child becomes allergic, and his or her allergies may be similar or different from your own.

CHAPTER 4

THE PRIMARY CHARACTERISTICS OF ALLERGIES

THREE IMPORTANT CONCEPTS are basic to the understanding of allergic reactions in the nose:

1. The Phases of an Allergic Reaction in the Nose
2. The Priming Effect
3. The Twitchy Nose

THE PHASES OF AN ALLERGIC REACTION IN THE NOSE

There are several phases through which an allergic reaction can pass in the causation of symptoms. For reasons that are not known, however, not all allergic reactions go through all phases. The phases through which an allergic reaction in your nose can evolve are as follows:

Phase I: The Early Nasal Response
Phase II: The Quiescent Phase
Phase III: The Late Nasal Response
Phase IV: The Hyperresponsive Phase
Phase V: The Delayed Nasal Response

Each phase occurs during a specific time period following exposure to an agent to which you are allergic, as will be discussed below. One, more than one, or all of these phases may be important to the development of your allergic rhinitis symptoms.

Phase I: The Early Nasal Response

The typical early nasal response begins within seconds of exposure to the allergy-causing substance with the onset of sneezing, runny nose, nasal congestion, and itching of the nose, throat, and palate. These symptoms peak rapidly, gradually clearing over a period of up to 2 hours (figure 4-1).

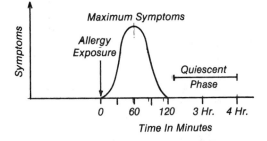

Figure 4-1: The Early Nasal Response

Phase II: The Quiescent Phase

Following the early nasal response is a period known as the quiescent phase. No significant symptoms occur during this phase (figure 4-1). Here, the mediators causing the early nasal response have been spent, and those that will cause the late nasal response are in the process of being formed and setting the stage for later phases.

Phase III: The Late Nasal Response

The late nasal response begins some 4 to 6 hours after exposure to the allergy-causing substance. A late response is not always preceded by an early response. Symptoms of the late response are similar to those experienced during the early response, but they reach the level of peak discomfort more slowly and persist for a longer period of time (figure 4-2). The late response seems to be driven primarily by mediators derived from the basophil cells. These mediators signal inflammatory cells-eosinophils and neutrophils-to enter the area. These cells then release their own unique set of chemical mediators into the tissue of the nasal mucosa. These mediators, in conjunction with those released by the basophil cells, cause both the recurrence of nasal symptoms as well as the development of an intense inflammatory reaction.

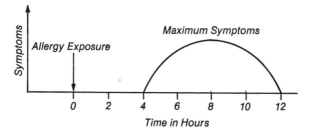

Figure 4-2: The Late Nasal Response

Phase IV: The Hyperresponsive Phase

Something very interesting happens to the nose after it has passed through the late nasal response: it becomes *more* responsive to *less* stimulation, hence the term *hyperresponsive* (figure 4-3). This hyperresponsiveness can be viewed from two separate perspectives: *priming* and *twitchiness*.

Priming. This term refers to a phenomenon that has long been observed by patients and physicians: as a pollen season progresses, patients can experience similar or worsening symptoms at lower levels of exposure (low pollen counts) than they had experienced earlier in the season with higher exposure (high pollen counts). In other words, late in a pollen season it takes less pollen in the air to initiate an allergic response than it did at the beginning of the season. Primed patients also note that they are more reactive to lower levels of exposure to other allergens: dusts, molds, mites, and animals.

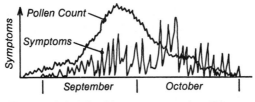

Figure 4-3: The Hyperresponsive Phase
Nasal "Priming" and Nasal "Twitchiness"

The Twitchy Allergic Nose. This term refers to an additional phenomenon observed by patients and physicians: the longer one seems to be bothered by allergic nasal symptoms, the more one's nose is "twitched," or symptoms are triggered by nonspecific, nonallergic factors. Some common categories of nonspecific, nonallergic factors include the following:

Aerosols	Chemicals
Pollutants	Bright lights
Smoke	Weather conditions
Powders	Newsprint
Cosmetics	

A combination of avoidance of allergens and twitching agents, medications to prevent the development of symptoms, medications to control symptoms once they've developed, and allergy desensitization injections can be used to control the results of the allergic nasal response. These are discussed in detail in chapters 10- 18.

Phase V: The Delayed Nasal Response

Some researchers believe that an additional, separate, and distinct response can be experienced between 24 and 96 hours after exposure to an allergy-causing substance and that either it can occur in conjunction with the early and/or late phase responses or it can be experienced as an independent response (figure 4-4). The symptoms are similar to those of the early and late responses.

The delayed response has not been subjected to as much study as have the early and late responses, so the "facts" of these limited observations await additional confirmation.

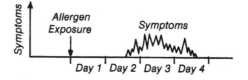

Figure 4-4: The Delayed Nasal Response

QUESTIONS AND ANSWERS

1. I get severe symptoms for about an hour after I've been exposed to cats, but I don't experience a recurrence of symptoms 4 to 6 hours after that. Since my allergy doesn't go through all the phases of a "normal" allergy reaction, are my symptoms coincidental but not allergic?

Your symptoms are most certainly allergic: you just have an early nasal response to cats, but not a late nasal response. As said above, you may not experience each of the possible phases of an allergic response. The truth is that most people do not experience each of these phases.

2. I seem to be bothered by my dust allergy only in the fall when my ragweed hay fever is a problem. Why is this so?

You are experiencing priming. As a pollen season progresses, it takes less exposure to the specific pollen allergen as well as other allergens to trigger symptoms. Your allergy to dust may not be sufficient to trigger your symptoms by itself, but, once your nose becomes hyperresponsive during ragweed season, it will become reactive to the dust that did not bother you before.

3. When I am exposed to cigarette smoke, my nose runs, stops up, and I occasionally sneeze. My doctor says that I'm not allergic to smoke, that it's just an irritant. I don't understand. I have the same symptoms to smoke as if I were allergic to it.

The nose has only a few symptoms with which it can respond to any stimulus, either allergen, irritant, or infectious. The symptoms caused by an irritant or infection may be similar to those caused by an allergen. What differs is the mechanism that causes the symptoms: an allergic reaction begins the process that results in allergic nasal symptoms; irritants stimulate your nose's nerve endings, which transmit signals to the brain, which then relays a message to your nose tissue to swell, run, or sneeze, etc. Infectious agents cause an inflammatory reaction, which causes changes in your nasal tissue, and you experience those changes as symptoms. The mechanism for smoke symptoms is a reflex. That for ragweed, for example, is allergic. That for the common cold, infectious. This will become more clear in chapter 8.

CHAPTER 5

THE POLLENS THAT CAUSE

SEASONAL ALLERGIC RHINITIS

TREE POLLENS, grass pollens, and weed pollens cause allergic nasal symptoms in millions of people. Pollen is that part of plants that contains the male genetic material. The units in which this material is held are called pollen grains. Two walls surround the genetic material in each grain. The innermost wall, the intine, is very thin and fragile. The outer protective wall, the exine, is relatively thick and highly resistant to destruction. Pollen grains from different plants look as different from one another as do the plants from which they come, a fact which is best appreciated when the grains are stained with special chemicals and viewed under a microscope. This is, in fact, what is done when a pollen count is made. Stained pollen grains are beautiful, intricate structures. For example, ragweed pollen resembles a golf ball, oak pollen an intergalactic starfighter, and cypress pollen, Pac Man.

Pollination is the term used to describe the transfer of pollen grains from the anther, the male organ of plants, to the stigma, the female organ of plants. Once transfer is completed, fertilization can take place. Surprisingly, only a small percentage of the thousands of plant pollens that exist are released into the air under circumstances sufficient to allow them to cause nasal allergy symptoms.

For a pollen to cause nasal allergies, it must meet four requirements:

- It must be produced in massive quantities.
- Its primary process of pollination must be via wind, not insects.
- It must be able to stimulate our immune system to produce an allergic response.
- We humans must be sufficiently exposed to the pollen to develop an allergy.

In order to be successfully wind pollinated, a plant and its pollen must have the following characteristics:

- A large number of pollen grains must be produced.
- The pollen must be aerodynamically sound, i.e., it must be of the right size, structure, and weight to be carried by the wind.
- The structure of the plant and its geographic location must favor the release of pollen into the wind.
- Pollen release during the season and during the day must be timed to optimize capture by the female organ.
- Like plants should be closely spaced to one another.

What a Pollen Count Can Tell You

A pollen count is simply that: a count of the average number of pollen grains contained in a cubic yard of air during the collection time, usually 24 hours.

Special devices have been developed to collect pollen and ensure an accurate count of the amount of pollen in a unit of air. Currently, the most commonly used method is that of specially coated glass rods. During predetermined time intervals, the rods are rotated in the air for specified intervals. As the rods are rotated, pollen grains from the air stick to the coated surface.

After 24 hours of such intermittent sampling (usually from

8 AM one morning until 8 AM the next morning) the rods are collected and stained. As the staining fluids are absorbed by the pollen grains, the grains distend and assume a highly characteristic appearance, one generally very different from that of the natural pollen. This change in appearance on staining permits most pollens to be easily identified. The pollen grains are then counted. The average number of grains of each pollen, as well as the average total number of pollen grains per cubic yard of air sampled, is then calculated as the pollen count for the last 24 hours.

When you hear about or read about today's pollen count, remember that that sample was taken from 8 AM yesterday until 8 AM today.

The amount of pollen in the air is affected by several factors. If you are following the pollen counts provided by the television, radio and/or print media in your area, it will be helpful for you to be aware of these variants:

1. The pollen count you hear or read about today is always **at least 24 hours old.**

2. **"Rain tends to wash pollen out of the air"** is generally a true statement: large droplets are not efficient pollen removers, but small droplets are very efficient. Therefore, brief thunderstorms are less efficient pollen removers than are prolonged gentle rains. In fact, thunderstorms may actually redisperse settled pollen in the air.

3. **Humidity** affects the pollination process. During times of high relative humidity, pollen grains tend to absorb moisture. This moisture adds weight and fills the tiny air pockets in the grains' outer walls, making them less aerodynamic. During periods of low relative humidity, water evaporates from the pollen grains walls. This opens the air pockets and lightens the pollen, making it more buoyant. This is why the combination of low humidity and a windy day increases the amount of pollen in the air—and increases the misery of allergy sufferers.

4. **Temperature** affects pollen counts. Warm air encourages the process of pollination, whereas cool temperatures reduce pollen production.

Which Pollens Cause Allergic Rhinitis?

The pollens of trees, grasses, and weeds account for 99.99 percent of all pollen-induced allergic rhinitis. Let's look at each type in more detail.

Tree Pollens. There are more than 50,000 species of trees worldwide. Some 600 to 700 of these are native to North America, but only the pollen from about 65 of these has been shown to cause allergic rhinitis. As you would expect, the trees causing symptoms are those most commonly found around and within inhabited areas.

Tree pollens generally show little cross reactivity: that is, in general, you must develop an allergy to each specific tree pollen in order for it to cause symptoms. However, there are two tree families that are exceptions: the family containing the alders, beeches, birches, and oaks, and the family of the junipers and cedars. With respect to these, if you are allergic to the pollen of one member of the family, you will probably experience symptoms from one or more other family members.

Grass Pollens. A grass is any member of the botanical family Gramineae, which contains some 4,500 species. However, the pollens of only a small percentage of the grasses— mostly members of the same subfamily—cause the majority of grass-induced allergic rhinitis. These do so because they are widely distributed and release enormous amounts of pollen into the air each season. These plants are so ubiquitous that none of us is safe from grass pollen anywhere in North America. Even in downtown New York City, you can become sufficiently exposed to grass pollen to develop allergic rhinitis.

The grasses to which people commonly become allergic are shown in table 5-1.

TABLE 5-1
Grass Pollens Causing Allergic Rhinitis

Grass	Area of North America Where Most Common
Bahia	South
Bermuda	South, Pacific Coast
Bluegrass	North, Canada
Fescue	North
Johnson	South
Orchard	North, Canada
Rye	North
Timothy	North, Canada
Sweet Vernal	Pacific Northwest
Red Top	North, Canada
Velvet	North, Pacific NW

Included in the grass family are the cereals (oats, barley, rice, corn, wheat). Most of the cereals have large, heavy pollens that can be carried on air currents only for very short distances, not the miles required of pollens that are going to cause widespread allergic reactions. Hence, grass pollen-allergic people are unlikely to be triggered by pollens from a cereal unless they are in proximity during the cereal's pollination.

Weed Pollens. A weed is simply a plant that grows where it's not wanted. Weeds release enormous amounts of pollen during pollen season, and thus serve as a major cause of allergic rhinitis. The weed pollens that cause allergic symptoms are listed in table 5-2.

The single most important family of weeds is that of the ragweeds (Compositea). Composed of some 20,000 species, ragweeds are similar to trees and grasses in that only a handful cause the majority of allergic rhinitis. These pollens are primarily a problem to residents of the warmer parts of the Western Hemisphere, although ragweed hay fever has been reported in limited regions of France, Russia, and the Balkan countries. Of note is that Africa, Australia, Europe, and Great Britain remain essentially ragweed free.

TABLE 5-2
Weed Pollens Causing Allergic Symptoms

Weed Family	Common Names of Weeds
Amaranths	Redroot pigweed
	Western water hemp
Chenopods	Russian thistle
	Burning bush
	Lambs quarters
Compositea	Ragweeds
Dock-knotwoods	Sheep sorrell
Nettles	Nettles
Plantains	Buckhorn plantain

The Pollen Seasons

In general, there are five different pollen seasons in North America (table 5-3).

The Early Spring Pollen Season. The early spring season begins in February and goes through March. The predominant pollens involved are those of trees.

The Late Spring Pollen Season. The late spring pollen season extends from April through June/July. The predominant late spring pollens are those of both trees and grasses.

TABLE 5-3
General Pollen Seasons for North America

Pollen	Ja	F	Mr	Ap	My	Je	Jl	Ag	S	O	N	D
Trees		✔	✔	✔	✔	✔	✔					✔
Grasses			✔	✔	✔	✔						
Weeds								✔	✔	✔		

The Summer Pollen Season. The summer pollen season begins in June and extends through August. The tree and grass pollens fade by mid summer, generally, and are followed closely by the late summer—fall weeds.

The Fall Pollen Season. The fall pollen season is the weed season, ragweed being the predominant weed pollen.

The Winter Pollen Season. The winter months in most areas of the country are typically pollen free. Exceptions do occur in south central Texas, Florida, and Southern California.

Knowing the Pollens of Importance in Your Region

In the United States and Canada, there are 10 distinct pollen regions, based on specific differences in the types of tree, grass, and weed pollens that are present as well as the onset, intensity, and duration of their pollination. Although sharp boundaries are shown on the map, in appendix I, there is significant overlap of pollens along the boundaries of adjacent areas.

The tables in appendix I provide details of the specific pollen seasons within these 10 pollen regions of the United States as well as of Hawaii, New Zealand, England and Australia.

QUESTIONS AND ANSWERS

1. I just found out that I'm allergic to elm pollen. Does that mean that the other tree pollens will trigger my allergy symptoms?

Elm pollen is unique and is unable to cross-react with any of the other tree pollens. As a result, other tree pollens will not cause symptoms because of your allergy to elm. If you begin having symptoms at times when elm pollen is not in the air, reconsult your allergist, as it is likely you have become allergic to another tree or to other types of pollen.

2. My friend says that she can't go to San Antonio from December through January because of the mountain cedar pol-

len. I didn't think that trees pollinated at that time of the year in Texas or anywhere else. Who is correct?

Your friend knows a lot about pollen. Although, in general, trees pollinate from the early spring to midsummer, in south central Texas, mountain cedar pollinates during December and January—and does so with a vengeance. This is an exception to the general rule that trees pollinate only in the spring.

3. I've heard that if you are allergic to grass, you shouldn't eat breakfast cereals (barley, oats, corn, wheat, rice), because these cereals are in the grass family and cross-react with grass pollen. Is this correct?

While cereals are in the grass family, breakfast cereals do not bother people who are grass allergic. Being allergic to pollen from the cereal plants does not necessarily mean that you will be allergic to the food grains produced by the plant. The situation is the same for pecans and pecan tree pollen. You can be allergic to the pollen and still enjoy the nut.

4. My hayfever is a problem just about the time that the goldenrod begins to pollinate, but my doctor told me that I couldn't be allergic to goldenrod. I don't understand.

In all likelihood you are actually allergic to ragweed pollen, which is the major airborne pollen at the time that goldenrod pollinates. You may not have noticed that the ragweeds are also pollinating at the same time as the goldenrods. They do not take on the bright gold color of the goldenrods so their pollen status is not as obvious. However, your doctor may be only partially correct. Ragweed and goldenrod are very closely related. If you are allergic to ragweed, it is highly likely that you will exhibit allergic symptoms if you are exposed to goldenrod. Still, because goldenrod pollen is quite heavy, it is normally carried by the wind only a few feet from its plant. Therefore, you would almost have to physically bump into the goldenrod plant to expose yourself sufficiently to its pollen to have symptoms. Although this seems unlikely, it can happen, as many a hiker and hunter can tell you.

CHAPTER 6

HOUSE DUST, HOUSE DUST MITES, MOLD SPORES, DOGS, CATS, AND OTHER CAUSES OF PERENNIAL ALLERGIC RHINITIS

PEOPLE WHO DO NOT HAVE allergic noses have no reason to think of house dust as anything other than a reason to change the bed, sweep and mop the floor, vacuum the carpet or hang a small carpet outside and beat on it with a stick. People with allergic rhinitis know otherwise. To them, house dust is a dirty trick.

HOUSE DUST?

The dust in your house is the sum of your environmental accumulations. It is a mixture that can include dried food particles, outside dust, pollen particles, mold spores, fibers, insect parts and droppings, pesticides, hair, shed skin cells, and dried saliva and urine from indoor pets.

What Is It In House Dust That Causes Allergies?

In laboratories around the world a debate has raged for years: Is there an allergen in house dust that is unique to dust, or are the symptoms caused by an allergy to one of the already—recognized agents comprising the dust—the most commonly suggested culprit being the house dust mite? Although the answer is not completely resolved to everyone's satisfaction, it appears that most allergic reactions to dust are due to an allergy to one of its constituents, most commonly the house dust mite. However, any of dust's constituents can be the cause of your symptoms: other insects and their droppings (most notably those of the cockroach), as well as animal (cat and dog) dander particles. Unfortunately, many allergic people are genetically disposed to react to more than one component of their house dust. They may, for example, react to mites, mold spores, pollens, and cat saliva.

How To Tell If You Are Allergic To House Dust

If when you vacuum, sweep, dust, and clean (or are present when this is done) you get a runny, itchy, stopped-up nose and a sneezing spell, you are probably allergic to something in house dust. The exact dust components causing your allergy can be determined by allergy testing, either of your skin or your blood serum.

If you are allergic to house dust, your symptoms tend to occur both in and out of the pollen seasons, are worse inside your home than outside, and seem to be more of a bother the longer you are indoors. It is common for dust-allergic symptoms to be worse on awakening in the mornings. Sleeping in a dusty bed or with a dusty pillow or bedding can contribute to your symptoms, as can the ceiling or oscillating fan that keeps the dust in your room suspended in the air while you sleep. Symptoms caused by something in house dust frequently lessen or clear when you go on vacation, then worsen when you return home.

HOUSE MITES

Although they are just one of many forms of insects with whom we share our living quarters, mites are the most important from an allergy perspective. A subclass of arachnids, two species of these microscopic creatures account for the majority of "house mite" allergies: *Dermatophagoides pteronyssinus* and *Dermatophagoides farinae* (figure 6- 1). One or both may be present in a home at any time. Cleanliness of the home or its occupants has nothing to do with their presence.

Mites need three things to survive: food, proper conditions of humidity, and safety. All three are found in homes. Their primary food source is shed skin cells from the human inhabitants and pets or feather-stuffed bedding and furniture. Skin shedding occurs in areas where humans spend the most time when at home, so there is good reason why the highest concentration of mites is found in stuffed furniture, carpeting, mattresses, and bedding. They also accumulate in clothing and stuffed toys.

The old saying "safe as a bug in a rug" should be the house mite motto. These microscopic creatures burrow deep into upholstered furniture, stuffed toys, bedding, and loose, long-pile carpet. Here, moisture conditions are optimal for survival and the mites are sufficiently protected so as to be impervious to vacuuming and other human efforts to eradicate them. Or, at least they *were*, as we will see below.

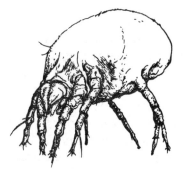

Figure 6-1: The House Dust Mite

Modern living—central heating, better sealed homes, and wall-to-wall carpeting—has benefited both man and mite. Mites require very specific conditions of humidity in relation to temperature for survival. Ideal conditions encompass a relative humidity of 55 to 75 percent over a temperature range of 59 to 95 degrees F. What better place than a home at 70 degrees F and a relative humidity of greater than 60 percent? Still, because temperature and humidity conditions vary greatly throughout the United States, the concentration of mites is greater in some areas than in others.

Mites have no lungs. They take air and water into their bodies primarily by diffusion through their shells. Thus, the greater the relative humidity, the greater their ability to acquire water. Their humidity needs are generally satisfied indoors, particularly in the winter months when the central heating system is functioning. In general, a combination of relative humidity of 40 to 50 percent and a temperature of 82 to 83 degrees F (28 to 34 degrees C) prohibits mite survival. So, whereas mites are found in most homes in the states bordering the east and gulf coasts, they occur in only a minority of homes in the states along the Rocky Mountains.

Humidifiers—Help Or Hindrance?

It is not a good idea for someone who is mite allergic to run a humidifier in an environment already sufficiently humid to support house mites, a condition common to millions of homes in the United States. Under these conditions room humidifiers are unlikely to significantly change the relative humidity of the air inside your home, usually do not produce particles of proper size to help either the nose or the lower airway, and they add moisture—a basic ingredient for mite survival—to your carpet, thus providing a water source for mites to live and breed. In addition, room humidifiers are rarely helpful to patients with nasal, sinus, bronchitis, or asthma problems.

To What Part Of The Mites Are People Allergic?

People are allergic to the mite fecal pellet. A single mite will produce some 200 times its weight in these potent, highly allergenic fecal pellets during its short lifetime (about 4 weeks). Once expelled, the pellets break down, incorporate into the dust of the house and become airborne when the carpet, bedding, furniture, and so on are disturbed. Microscopic in size, these particles are easily inhaled into the nose and lungs, where they trigger allergy symptoms. The density of the live mite population in your home determines the degree of problem you will have with mite fecal particles. Although dead mites and their body parts do become airborne, they do not contribute significantly to mite allergy.

THE MOLDS

A mold is a tiny member of the group of plants we call fungi. These are plants that lack a definite root and stem and have no leafy structures. Molds contain no chlorophyl and are composed of multiple, microscopic branching threads. Because they lack chlorophyll molds depend upon other plants and animal materials for nourishment.

Molds As Causes Of Allergic Rhinitis

Allergy-causing molds reproduce by forming microscopic spores that are then widely distributed by currents of air. It is to these airborne mold spores that we become allergic. In the air, the behavior of mold spores is very similar to that of pollens. Molds are common additions to outdoor and indoor air, and *mold counts*, like pollen counts, are commonly performed on outdoor air using special gathering devices.

Molds' ability to disperse on air currents depends upon a range of temperature, humidity, and wind conditions somewhat similar to that of the pollens. For example, certain mold spores settle with rain and increased humidity, only to rise again into the air with drying and increased wind. Others depend upon a rising humidity and rain droplets to release them into the air.

Molds differ from pollens in that, in general, they do not enter and exit the air with seasonal regularity. In other words, with a few very specific and localized exceptions, there isn't any "mold season" as there is a ragweed season. Molds tend to be in the outdoor air most of the year—from early spring until (and even after) the first frost. In general, however, mold counts are the highest in the warmer summer months (figure 6-2).

Like trees, grasses, and weeds, only a few of the many types of molds have been shown to cause allergic rhinitis. In fact, just four molds—*Alternaria, Aspergillus, Hormodendrum,* and *Penicillium*—account for most mold-induced allergic rhinitis. *Alternaria* and *Hormodendrum* are prominent outdoor molds. *Aspergillus* and *Penicillium* are common indoor molds. Penicillium is that green fuzzy stuff sometimes seen in homes. That dark, fuzzy stuff that may grow on the refrigerator walls or on foods such as bread or onions is another allergy-causing mold known as *Rhizopus.*

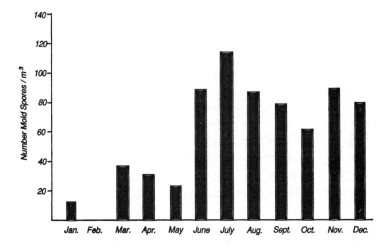

Figure 6-2: Moldspores: A Problem All Year

Where Do These Molds Tend To Grow?

Molds can grow and reproduce almost anywhere. It is not difficult for them to find suitable conditions of light, temperature, and humidity. Indoors, they may grow on floors, carpets, bedding, mattresses, and pillows (especially foam rubber), basements, food products, garbage pails, refrigerator drip-pans, humidifiers and air conditioning systems, wall paper, paints, plastics, flowers, soiled upholstery, wool clothing, old books and magazines, fruits, berries, and bathroom tile. Outdoors, molds commonly grow on garage dust, rotting or decaying vegetation, fresh cut grass, piles of leaves, rotting wood, compost piles, pasture grass, melons, peas, bananas, cotton, tomatoes, corn, sweet potatoes, mushrooms, hay bales, and areas of deep shade. The cutting of grass, raking of leaves, and thrashing and baling of hay can launch millions of mold particles into the air. These settle on your clothing and are carried into your home.

How To Tell If You Are Allergic To Molds

There are several clues. First, molds are a common cause of year-around allergic nasal symptoms. Another clue would be a flare-up of symptoms during the summer months when there is relatively little pollen but much mold in the air. Also suggestive are symptoms that worsen in the late fall after the ragweed has cleared from the air. In addition, symptoms that worsen during activities in areas where molds tend to grow and reproduce suggest molds as a possible allergen.

Food Cautions For Mold Sensitive People

Some people who are sensitive to airborne molds may react if those same molds are ingested. Table 6-1 lists the common foods and beverages that may contain molds or mold products that could trigger nasal or other allergic symptoms in mold-allergic patients. Foods developed by fermentation, meats, aged cheeses, and foods whose shelf lives are relatively long are the most likely to be mold contaminated. If you suspect that the ingestion of these or any other foods causes any type of symptom, nasal or other, you should avoid them and discuss your suspicion with your physician or allergist.

TABLE 6-1
Foods and Beverages That May Cause
Symptoms in Mold-Allergic People

Alcoholic beverages, especially beer and wine
Beets
Buttermilk
Breads: especially coffee cakes, pumpernickel
Catsup
Cheese, especially stored, aged, blue, cottage
Chile sauce
Cider and home-made root beer
Corned beef
Dried fruits: apricots, dates, figs, prunes, raisins
Frankfurters
Fish: pickled and smoked
Juices, canned
Mayonnaise
Meats: pickled and smoked
Mushrooms
Olives
Pickles
Pickled tongue
Relishes
Salad dressings
Sauerkraut
Sausage
Sour Cream
Tomatoes, especially canned
Vinegar and vinegar-containing foods

Mold Exposure Is Increased In Certain Occupations

Some people in certain occupations are at risk for increased mold-spore exposure, and hence the development of mold-spore allergy. Examples of these are shown in table 6-2:

TABLE 6-2
Types of Occupations at Risk for
Increased Mold-Spore Exposure

Bakers	Gardeners
Brewers	Mattress makers
Butchers	Mill workers
Carpenters	Paper/Books handlers
Cheese workers	Paper hangers
Farmers	Pharmaceutical workers
Florist	Plant nursery workers, landscapers
Furriers	

What you can do to reduce your exposure to mold spores will be discussed in chapter 10.

CATS

The exact incidence of cat allergy has not been established, but in my own practice it is one of the five most common allergens. Allergies to birds, gerbils, hamsters, and rabbits occur, although much less frequently than allergy to cat. Their exact incidence is likewise not clearly established.

If you are a cat-allergic person, you are well aware of the sneezing, nasal congestion, and runny nose that can occur within a few minutes of entering a home inhabited by a house cat. The substance responsible for these symptoms is a protein allergists refer to as *Fel d I* (this protein is the *1*st allergen *d*erived from *Fel*ines). Derived primarily from cat salivary glands and sebaceous (oil) glands of hair roots, Fel d I is primarily distributed by cat saliva and dander (material common to the superficial skin). Cat urine and feces contribute little to Fel d I's load in homes.

Easily airborne, Fel d I appears to remain so for hours, even in an undisturbed house (a house with no one in it). Walking on carpet or sitting on furniture containing this protein causes significant amounts of it to be released into the air. A protein of relatively low molecular weight, it can easily lodge in the nose and eyes or evade nasal entrapment and find its way into the lungs, thus wreaking misery upon cat-allergic family members or guests. As will be seen in chapter 10, it will take months for the cat allergen to abate from your home even after the cat itself has been banished to the outdoors.

DOGS

Like cats, dogs are common causes of perennial allergic rhinitis. The exact nature of the dog's allergenic proteins responsible for symptoms has not been delineated to the degree that that of cats and house mites has been. We do know that the allergens are proteins and that they are found primarily in the dog's shed skin and saliva. They also are found in dog hair, blood serum, urine, and feces, but these are not the sources of our primary exposure.

Myths About Allergy to Cats and Dogs

The First Myth: "I'm Not Allergic to My Dog, But I Can't Get NearMyNeighbor'sDog." This is a comment usually made by people whose dog lives inside, and in close relationship with them. The observation is partially true: such a person may not notice that her symptoms are triggered by her dog. However, the fact that she does not notice them doesn't mean that she isn't allergic to her dog.

Dog-allergic people whose pets live indoors frequently have daily symptoms that wax and wane in severity. Such people either cannot identify anything specific that triggers symptoms, or they tend to perceive that "everything" causes symptoms. The truth is, their symptoms have become a daily affair: They are exposed to dog allergen many hours out of each day because their dog lives indoors.

When this dog owner goes to her neighbor's home, she becomes exposed to a different amount of dog allergen. If this exposure is more intense than what she gets from her own dog, she will experience a flare-up of symptoms. To her, it seems as if she is allergic to the neighbor's dog and not her own, when, in truth, she is actually allergic to both her pet and her neighbor's. The increased degree of exposure to dog allergen at her neighbor's accounts for her increased symptoms while there.

The Second Myth: Short-Hair Dogs or Cats Cause Fewer Allergy Problems Than Their Long-Haired Counterparts. Remember this: *Dogs is Dogs! Cats is Cats!*

Also, as discussed above and in contrast to popular belief, dog and cat hair are far less important as causes of allergic symptoms than are *shed skin cells* and *saliva*. Therefore, don't judge the allergy-causing ability of a dog or cat by the length of its hair.

The Final Myth: "I'm Allergic to Cocker Spaniels But Not to Labradors." This statement implies that you can be allergic to one *breed* of dog, but not to another. This isn't true, although it may seem to be. Be aware that some breeds of dog either shed more "doggy" allergen in their skin and saliva than do other breeds, or they simply shed a greater volume of skin cells and saliva. Either results in a greater exposure to allergen from one breed than another, and therefore, in more allergic symptoms. But doggy allergen is doggy allergen; it is not unique to any breed. If you hang around the breed you think you are not allergic to long enough, you will eventually expose yourself sufficiently to develop symptoms.

OTHER ALLERGENS CAUSING PERENNIAL ALLERGIC RHINITIS

Other Mammals

Although they are not major constituents of modern home furnishings, horse hair and cow hair were at one time used as stuffing in furniture and mattresses, as well as in mattings, padding, and felts. Exposure to these allergens can still occur via older beds, carpets, carpet pads, chairs, and sofas.

Feathers

Although it is possible to be allergic to feathers, what we call our "allergy to feathers" is most likely a reaction to the house mites living in the feather pillows, not to the feathers themselves. Remember, feathers are specialized extensions of the skin of birds and are thus composed of epithelial cells, the basic foodstuff of house mites. As a rule, the older the feather pillow, the more of a problem it will present to an allergic person, due to the accumulation of mites over time. A feather pillow is such a perfect environment that a house mite couple finding their way into a feather pillow would no doubt think they'd died and gone to heaven.

Caution: We tend to forget that feathers are used in things other than pillows. Watch out for things like comforters, quilts, down jackets, and sleeping bags.

A Myth About Feathers: "I Can't Take Egg-Containing Vaccines Because I'm Allergic to Feathers." Horsefeathers! A reaction to feathers has nothing to do with eggs. Egg protein has to do with eggs. If you are truly allergic to eggs, you should take egg-grown vaccines only with great caution, if at all.

Cottonsead

This is one of the most potent allergens for humans. The culprit is a water soluble protein that is used most extensively in fertilizers and animal feeds. It can cause explosive symptoms when those allergic to it are exposed.

For the record, it is extremely unlikely that *cottonseed oil* contains any active cottonseed allergen, due to its extensive preparation process.

Kapok

Kapok is a light, cottonlike fiber derived from the fruit of the kapok tree, indigenous to Ceylon, India, Indonesia, the Philippines, and South America. After the fruit of the kapok tree is picked, workers remove the seeds and fibers and dry them in the sun. The fibers are lightweight, buoyant, and do not absorb water. It is these qualities that make it useful as a stuffing for mattresses, pillows, sleeping bags, and lifejackets. Like feather pillows, as it ages, it increases as a problem for allergic people, a characteristic some believe is due to its gradual invasion by house mites. Hence, kapok pillows should not replace feather pillows for feather-allergic people.

QUESTIONS AND ANSWERS

1. I'm allergic to Penicillium *mold. Does this mean that I'm also allergic to penicillin?*

No, it doesn't. The two are independent of one another. The reason for this is that when you are allergic to the mold *Penicillium*, you are allergic to a specific protein that it contains. Penicillin allergy involves an entirely different chemical, the drug penicillin or one of its metabolic products. These two allergies are no more related to one another than an allergy to ragweed pollen is related to an allergy to oak pollen.

2. If I am mold allergic, do I have to remove the potted plants from my home?

No, you don't. Potted plants in the home have been shown to raise the mold level in the home only very slightly. Expend your mold controlling energies in the areas of your home where they are most needed: bed, carpet, kitchen, bathroom, basement, etc. See chapter 10 for details.

3. I'm allergic to my cat, but do I really have to get rid of her?

The best treatment for an allergy to any animal is avoidance. If you have an inside cat, one option is to convert it to an outside pet and have minimal contact with it. This is difficult for people who have had an inside pet that has been "a part of the family" for years. In addition, sometimes the pet cannot adjust to being outdoors. The other option is to find the pet a new home. Cat allergen is difficult to control because it is very, very light and will float all over the house. So, even if you confine your cat to one or two rooms, the cat allergen will find its way throughout your home.

4. Is it true that if I am allergic to feathers I shouldn't eat chicken?

No, it isn't true. Reactions to feather allergens have nothing to do with chicken meat. Remember that almost all "feather allergies" are due not to feathers but to house mites.

CHAPTER 7

OCCUPATIONAL RHINITIS: ARE YOU ALLERGIC TO YOUR WORK?

OCCUPATIONAL RHINITIS refers to nasal symptoms caused or triggered by exposure to an agent in the workplace. This takes two forms:

Office Rhinitis: Symptoms occur in a particular office, or office building.
Nonoffice Rhinitis: Symptoms occur only in a special work situation.

Occupational rhinitis can affect a broad range of workers: the president of the company, the secretarial staff, the janitorial service, security, the gardener, as well as beauticians, photographers, and veterinarians.

There are only a few scientific studies that have determined the frequency with which workers in offices and office buildings suffer various symptoms. These studies suggest that from 15 to 35 percent of office workers have work related symptoms. There are many studies that have examined the frequency of development with which workers in nonoffice environments develop work-related symptoms. The focus of studies on the nonoffice occupations rather than office occupations stems from the interest in the unique agents to which these workers are exposed while on the job. These nonoffice occupation studies have shown that 20 to 30 percent of animal-laboratory workers become allergic to the animals with which they work, 10 percent of bakers become allergic to flour, and 30 percent of workers exposed to platinum salts will become allergic to these chemicals.

General Symptoms of Occupational Rhinitis

Congestion	Runny nose
Sneezing	Itchy nose, throat, palate
Burning or stinging	Headache
of the nose	Drainage and cough
Dry throat	

Office Rhinitis

The Causes of Office Rhinitis. Office rhinitis is occupational rhinitis caused by something in the *office* environment. The possible causes of office rhinitis are extensive. Common causes include inadequate ventilation of the workspace, cigarette smoke, chemical odors (cleaning agents, shampoos, insecticides, new furniture or carpeting), and indoor allergens, particularly dust mites and mold spores. Table 7-1 lists the more common causes of office rhinitis as well as their likely sources.

The Sick Building Syndrome. A special word about this problem is in order. Since the mid-1960s there has been a trend in the construction of office buildings toward tighter buildings. These are buildings in which the natural flow of air is impeded and is replaced by the mechanical control of ventilation. The sealed windows, prefabricated components, reduced ventilation rates are characteristics of modern construction, which when coupled with the trapping of chemicals, particles, odors (including smoke), and common indoor allergens create an unhealthy environment for many workers.

TABLE 7-1
Common Causes of Office Rhinitis

Causal Agent	Source(s)
Allergens	Dust mite, cockroach droppings, mold spores
Carbon monoxide	Tobacco smoke, gas range, space heaters, back drafting of water heaters or furnace, attached garages
Formaldehyde	Carpet, fabrics, fiberboard, fabrics, plywood, carpet
NO_2	Gas ranges, space heaters, furnaces
Particles in the air	Tobacco smoke, outside air, air from adjacent offices
Smoke	Cigarettes, cigars, pipes
Volatile organic compounds	Outgasing from paints, solvents, cleaning agents, glues, photocopiers
Semivolatile organic compounds	Insecticides

Add to the above situation an event such as a fire, a water leak, the laying of new carpet, the shampooing of old carpet, the waxing of floors, etc., and many workers can become symptomatic. This is called Sick Building Syndrome, Tight Building Syndrome, or Building-Related Illness. Rhinitis symptoms as well as eye irritation, cough, chest tightness, headache, and malaise can occur. Often, the only remedy required is to improve the ventilation in the office spaces involved so that harmful particles and odors are better removed.

Nonoffice Rhinitis

Table 7-2 lists some of the unique work situations in which exposure to an allergen or an irritant can cause nonoffice occupational rhinitis.

TABLE 7-2
Special Work Situations and Occupational Rhinitis

Occupation	Agent(s) Causing Symptoms
Aluminum handler	Aluminum Dust
Animal worker	Urine, dander (skin), blood, hair
Baker, miller, grain worker	Flour, grain dust, insects
Beauticians	Dyes, formalin, fluorocarbons
Beekeepers	Bee dust
Bookbinders	Glues
Cement workers	Cromium and cobalt
Coffee workers	Dust from green coffee beans
Detergent industry	Bacteria
Dockworkers	Grain weevils
Farmers	Soybean dust, grain dust, animals
Longshoremen	Coffee dust, grain dust
Meat wrappers, grocers	Polyvinylchloride
Pesticide workers	Organophosphates
Refinery workers	Platinum salts and acids
Textile workers	Cotton flax, jute, hemp
Welders	Stainless steel fumes
Wood workers	Wood dusts

The Two Most Common Ways That Occupational Agents Cause Rhinitis

1. **Irritant Reactions:** Agents that irritate the membrane of our noses are the most common causes of office rhinitis. At the top of the list of such agents is cigarette smoke.
2. **Allergic Reactions:** This is the most common mechanism of nonoffice rhinitis. As shown in table 7-2, longshoremen, farmers, veterinarians, and cement workers all can become allergic to agents unique to their workplaces.

When To Suspect Occupational Rhinitis

If you do not know or suspect a specific agent at work as a cause of your symptoms, here are five clues that suggest that something in your office is causing or contributing to your rhinitis, and that you should take a closer look at your workplace:

1. Your symptoms worsen at work.
2. Your symptoms are least bothersome at home.
3. Your symptoms are worse at the end of the work week than at its beginning.
4. When you are away from work for extended periods, such as weekends or vacations, you feel much better or clearer.
5. More than one-third of your co-workers suffer similar symptoms.

Resolving Occupational Rhinitis

1 . Do your best to identify the cause(s).
2. Once the cause is identified, eliminate or correct it. In most cases this is not difficult to do (see step 4). The most difficult task is to first recognize that a work-related problem exists.
3. Enlist the help of your boss or supervisor if necessary.
4. If you are unable to identify a cause, it would be wise to have the air exchange in your office checked. Frequently, simply improving the exchange of air in your workplace will greatly improve symptoms. The same people who service your air conditioning-heating system either should be able to do this or can advise you of whom to call.
5. At this time, the expense involved in consulting someone skilled in the measurement of particles, smoke, and various chemicals in your environment is futile, since almost none of them are equipped to confirm any suspicions that might be uncovered in such a study.

A Word About Smoking vs. Not Smoking In Offices

Because cigarette smoke is such a common cause of office rhinitis, a few comments on the rights of smokers vs. the rights of nonsmokers are in order. This is an issue that has not been settled, but whose face is changing. Here is the current situation:

• There is no national law regarding smoking in general. Smoking is limited to designated areas in federal buildings and is prohibited on certain domestic airline flights.

• It is possible through state and local ordinances to prohibit smoking in public buildings, as well as permit businesses to restrict or prohibit smoking, whichever they deem in the best interest of their employees.

• The smokers' defense regarding restrictions to their right to smoke in the workplace has been that they had as much right to smoke as nonsmokers had to not smoke, and that they could exercise this right when and where they wished, respecting safety factors and local ordinances.

• However, a recent declaration by the Surgeon General of the United States declared that cigarette smoke was harmful to nonsmokers who inhaled that smoke, the so-called passive smoker. It is my understanding that this declaration offers the potential for further legal limitation of the rights of smokers: although smokers still have the right to smoke, they do not have the right to harm the health of those around them. Since smoke from the tip of their cigarette as well as that which they exhale pollutes the air that others must breathe, and since breathing such second-hand smoke has been declared harmful, it is quite possible that their right to smoke in an environment in which nonsmokers work or play will not be upheld. This has yet to be tested in court, but it is my guess that such a test is only a matter of time.

The Future: More Research Is Needed

The serious study of agents in the office environment that cause occupational rhinitis and other medical conditions is just beginning. The definition of which agents are important as causes of symptoms and at what levels of exposure they cause symptoms as well as the clarification of how exposure can be limited are needed. During the next 10 years the scientific studies required to resolve these issues should be well underway.

The results of these studies should bring forth information that can then be translated into making the workplace, both office and nonoffice, a more healthy environment.

QUESTIONS AND ANSWERS

1. We had a problem with workers' noses burning and becoming stuffed up at the office in which I work. It was corrected by improving our ventilation system. Is this common?

This is one of the most common observations made by workers who correct problems in offices. Often, all that is required in an environment that is "stale" is to increase the circulation of air throughout the environment.

2. I read somewhere that if you are cat allergic and several people who work in the same office own cats, you could have nasal symptoms at work from the "cat" they bring to work on their clothes. Is this true?

Yes, it is. Over a period of time, these cat owners can bring enough cat allergen to work to cause you to have symptoms. There is a test that can be performed on the vacuumed dust from your workplace that can determine whether or not there is enough cat allergen in your office environment to cause trouble. If you suspect that this is a problem, ask your doctor about the test.

3. Is there a test for dust mites as well?

Yes, there is. Your doctor should know about this as well.

PART THREE

Conditions That Masquerade As Allergic Rhinitis

CHAPTER 8

IF IT'S NOT AN ALLERGY, WHAT IS IT?

IS THIS STATEMENT True or False?

"If it isn't a cold, it must be an allergy." It is False. The fact is that there are more than 20 different nonallergic conditions that your doctor will consider when determining the cause(s) for your allergy-like nasal symptoms, each one discussed in this chapter.

Doctors are trained to consider all of the possibilities for each of your symptoms so that they can accurately differentiate one cause of your symptoms from another, ultimately reaching the correct cause or diagnosis. This process is called *differential diagnosis*. This chapter is about the differential diagnosis of allergic rhinitis. It is about all of those things that can cause symptoms similar to those of allergic rhinitis but that are not allergic rhinitis.

Important: Remember that it is quite possible for you to have *more than one type* of rhinitis. Several types may even occur at the same time. Example: let's say you are suffering with fall hay fever, and on top of this you have caught a cold, and on top of that you have been using nasal decongestant sprays 4 to 5 times per day for the last two weeks to keep your nose open. You have three different types of rhinitis contributing to your symptoms, all at the same time: seasonal allergic rhinitis (the hay fever), infectious rhinitis (the cold), and chemical rhinitis (the overuse of over-the-counter (OTC) nasal decongestant sprays). It is important for you to be aware that there may be multiple causes of your nasal symptoms. This awareness will help you eliminate any confusion about your symptoms, help you seek and obtain treatment in a more timely and effective manner, and enable you to better understand that treatment.

Conditions That Masquerrade As Allergic Rhinitis

Table 8-1 lists the most common conditions that might cause symptoms similar to allergic rhinitis. It is helpful to think about them in terms of which ones are really due to allergies (the allergic rhinitis syndromes) and which ones are not (the nonallergic rhinitis syndromes). The **nonallergic rhinitis syndromes** subdivide into those caused by some kind of anatomical abnormality, the **anatomic syndromes,** and those not due to abnormal anatomy, the **Nonanatomic Syndromes.** The anatomic syndromes then break down into those that generally cause nasal congestion as their main symptom, the **congestion syndromes,** and those that generally cause runny nose as their main symptom, the **rhinorrhea syndromes.** The table below should clarify the causes of rhinitis.

THE NONALLERGIC RHINITIS SYNDROMES

Nonallergic rhinitis takes many forms: the common cold, being "hooked" on OTC nasal decongestant sprays, or having a deviated nasal septum are all examples of a condition that is not allergic, but can cause symptoms that are similar to allergic nasal symptoms. Believe it or not, more people suffer from nonallergic rhinitis than from allergic rhinitis: 60 percent of all people who suffer with nasal problems do so because of one or another form of *nonallergic rhinitis.*

Table 8-1: 24 Different Causes of Allergic-Like Symptoms

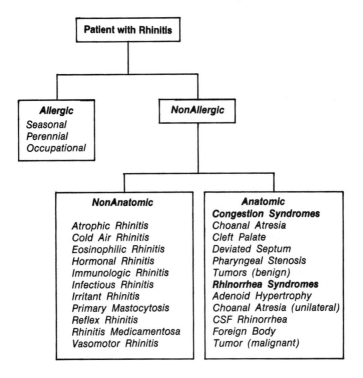

How can I tell if my nose trouble is nonallergic? Your doctor will be able to tell you this. His or her answer will be based on the following:

First, as your doctor will ask the many detailed questions required to obtain a detailed medical history about your nose, both of you will become aware, through your answers, that the things you recognize as triggers of your nasal symptoms are not allergy things—like pollens, dusts, mold spores, or pets—but nonallergy things—like odors, smells, weather changes, and infection. I have included such a history for you to complete in chapter 9.

Second, in contrast to allergic rhinitis, your symptoms will not tend to occur only during the pollen seasons in your area.

(The pollen seasons are discussed in chapter 5 and a tabular guide to them is included in appendix 1.)

Third, your allergy tests will reveal no positive reactions to any airborne allergen (dust, molds, mite, animals, occupational agents, or pollens).

NonAnatomic Conditions Masquerading As Allergic Rhinitis

This group of illnesses includes those disorders that are not due either to allergic causes or to some abnormality of the anatomy of the nose.

Atrophic Rhinitis. More common in women for reasons that are not clear, this is a disorder in which the lining of the nose becomes chronically inflamed and thinned and large numbers of scabs accumulate on the lining membrane of the nose. Patients with this problem are most bothered by two symptoms: a characteristic sensation of nasal congestion in spite of a wide-open nasal passageway, and a foul odor, called ozena, that comes from the nose. Ozena is caused by a bacterial infection of the lining of the nose.

Atrophic rhinitis is uncomfortable to have and difficult to treat. The cause of atrophic rhinitis is not known, although a causative role for bacteria, chemical fumes, cigarette smoke, and viral agents all have been suggested.

Cold Air Rhinitis. You've probably walked down a cold, windy street and experienced mild nasal congestion, runny nose, and occasional sneezing. This is such a common experience that most of us consider it to be normal. However, some people experience severe nasal symptoms on exposure to cold air. In these people, mast cells release the same mediators that they would if the person had been exposed to something to which they were allergic, causing these people to experience symptoms very similar to severe allergic rhinitis. However, this is not an allergy because cold is not an allergen and no IgE antibodies are involved.

Eosinophilic Nonallergic Rhinitis (E-NAR) Syndromes.
When a physician makes a smear of your nasal mucus to examine under a microscope, he or she is looking to see what type(s) of cells are present as a means of differentiating one form of rhinitis from another. The eosinophil, a red-staining cell easily seen in nasal smears, is one cell doctors always look for. Although common in each of the three types of allergic rhinitis and frequently called "allergy cells," they also appear in the nasal mucus of a group of nonallergic rhinitis syndromes called the eosinophilic nonallergic rhinitis syndromes (E-NAR syndromes).

The symptoms of E-NAR syndromes are no different from those of the other forms of nonallergic rhinitis, and can include nasal congestion, runny nose, and sneezing. These syndromes are likely to be seen in patients who also happen to suffer from asthma, chronic sinus infections, nasal polyps, or have severe reactions to aspirin.

While only your doctor can distinguish the subtleties between one form of eosinophilic rhinitis from another, you should be aware that these forms of nasal dysfunction exist and can be identified by a nasal smear. It is also important that you and your doctor know that a nasal smear full of eosinophils does not always mean that you are allergic, a misconception held by many physicians and patients.

Hormonal/Endocrine Rhinitis. Rhinitis can result from an imbalance in either thyroid hormones or male/female sexual hormones.

• **Hypothyroidism:** Some patients with an underfunctioning thyroid gland experience nasal symptoms. Their predominant symptom is nasal congestion.

• **Sex Hormones:** Many women experience annoying nasal symptoms, particularly nasal congestion, when various sex hormone levels are increased, such as during pregnancy, ovulation, or while taking birth control pills. Both men and women may experience nasal congestion and runny nose during sexual excitation.

Immunologic Nasal Disease. Normally, our immune system helps protect our nose against infection. As such, nasal symptoms can occur as a complication of the improper functioning of one's immune system. Symptoms can include any of those associated with abnormal nose function: congestion, runny nose, sneezing, drainage, bleeding, loss of sense of smell, and foul odors.

Infectious Rhinitis. We have all had this type of rhinitis: the common cold. It is caused by infection from one of hundreds of viruses. Viruses, like bacteria, are microscopic organisms. However, they are much smaller than bacteria, and unlike most bacteria, they are incapable of growth and reproduction outside of living cells. Hence, they live in our cells as parasites. Viral infections account for 90 percent of all cases of infectious rhinitis.

The common cold usually begins with a sore throat, then quickly progresses to include runny nose, increased postnasal drainage, nasal congestion, sniffling, and sneezing. It generally lasts 7 to 14 days and is commonly associated with a sensation of fatigue, a low-grade fever, enlarged lymph nodes in the neck, some general achiness, and reduced appetite.

Unappreciated is the fact that it is normal for children to have up to five colds each year. Almost equally unappreciated is the fact that many children in day-care environments will have many more colds per year than this, simply because of their increased exposure.

Bacterial infections can cause infectious rhinitis, but they do so in only about 10 percent of all cases. Bacteria are microscopic organisms, larger than viruses, and generally capable of maintaining their life outside of living cells. They are common causes of ear infections, sinus infections, and pneumonia.

Irritant Rhinitis. In this form of rhinitis, symptoms result from exposure to irritants: various types of dusts and chemical fumes, such as perfume, hair sprays, carpet fresheners, gasoline, and chemical pollutants. If you have this form of rhinitis, your symptoms can include nasal congestion, runny nose, and sneezing.

Primary Nasal Mastocytosis. This is a rare form of rhinitis that is characterized by an accumulation of an enormous number of mast cells in the lining membrane of the nose. These cells release chemicals that induce nasal symptoms. Chronic runny nose and nasal stuffiness are typical. The good side of this form of rhinitis is that it is not associated with asthma, the formation of nasal polyps (see below), or recurring episodes of infected sinuses.

Reflex Rhinitis. Reflexes can cause significant nasal symptoms. Those reflexes that can cause rhinitis are listed in table 8-2.

TABLE 8-2
Reflexes Causing Nasal Symptoms

Reflex Stimulus	Nasal Symptoms(s)
Eye (bright light)	Sneezing
Lying on your side	Congestion on that side of nose
Body cooling	Congestion
Anxiety	Congestion
Fear	Decongestion
Exertion	Decongestion
Eating	Runny nose, sneezing

Rhinitis Medicamentosa. This term defines nasal symptoms (rhinitis) caused by a medication you are taking (medicamentosa) to help some other medical problem (like high blood pressure). The most common symptom of rhinitis medicamentosa is nasal congestion, but runny nose, burning, bleeding, and a sensation of dryness in the nose may occur.

There are two general types of rhinitis medicamentosa:

• **Local Rhinitis Medicamentosa—"The Nose Drop Nose"** — is caused by medications you are placing in your nose. Some examples include OTC nasal decongestant drops, sinus sprays, and cocaine. OTC nose drops or sprays used to unstop a congested nose are good news/bad news drugs. The good news is that they do unstop noses. The bad news is that if you use them for too long (more than about 5 to 7 days), they tend to "rebound." This means that after opening the nose for a short time, they cause the lining of the nose to swell, thus stopping the nose up once again. Then, you use the spray to reopen your nose and it opens for a short time, but the swelling closes it again. At this point you are hooked on nose sprays or drops. All available OTC nasal decongestant sprays and drops will cause this rebound effect, so use them sparingly. It is likely that you are becoming hooked on nasal sprays if you cannot stop them after 5 to 7 days or find that your nasal congestion is worsening in spite of their use. If this happens, call your doctor. He or she can recommend medications which will stop this rebound effect.

• **Systemic Rhinitis Medicamentosa—"The Iatrogenic Nose"**—is caused by medications you are taking by mouth for other illnesses. Some examples include Accutane for acne and some blood pressure medications. The term *iatrogenic* refers to an unfavorable response to treatment caused by the treatment itself. The term *systemic* refers to the entire person, in contrast to a single part of a person, such as the nose. Systemic medications exert their effect throughout the body and have the potential of affecting any organ. Topical medications work only where they are placed (nose sprays work only in the nose). The term *the iatrogenic nose* refers to nasal symptoms that are caused by medications taken for medical conditions other than nasal problems.

Systemic rhinitis medicamentosa results from a medication you are taking for some other problem. Like local rhinitis medicamentosa, its most common symptom is nasal congestion. The most common types of medications causing this are those for high blood pressure, such as those containing bydralazine, guanethidine, methyldopa, prazosin, and reserpine. These medications dilate blood vessels in the body, including the nose, and this causes nasal congestion. Other medications taken systemically can cause nasal symptoms. Table 8-3 lists by brand-name commonly prescribed medications that contain ingredients that can cause nasal symptoms as well as the type(s) of symptoms they can cause. Keep in mind that most of these medications cause nasal symptoms only in a small percentage of patients who use them. If your nasal symptoms began or worsened after you started taking a medication, talk with your doctor about the possibility of its contributing to your nasal symptoms.

A more detailed listing of the medications taken by mouth that can cause nasal symptoms is found in appendix II.

Vasomotor Rhinitis. Last on the list of nonallergic, nonanatomic rhinitis syndromes is vasomotor rhinitis. It is last on this list because it is a diagnosis of exclusion, reached only after each of the other possible causes discussed above have been eliminated. Its nasal symptoms are similar to those of allergic and nonallergic rhinitis.

How one treats the variety of nasal symptoms that result from allergic as well as nonallergic, nonanatomic rhinitis is discussed in detail in chapters 10-18.

Anatomic Causes of Chronic NonAllergic Rhinitis

In searching for the cause of your nasal symptoms, always keep in mind that if the internal anatomy of the nose is not normal, symptoms can result. Anatomical aberrations can be genetic or can be caused by some disease or injury since birth.

Anatomic Causes of a NonAllergic Stuffy Nose

If you or your child have a chronically stuffy nose, you may have one of the five disorders listed below. All are correctable using modern surgical procedures.

Deviated Nasal Septum. The wall that divides the inside of our nose into right and left sides is called the nasal septum (septum means a partition). If this wall is crooked, i.e., if it encroaches on one side of the nose or the other, it is called a *deviated* (off course) *septum.* If the septum deviates too much, it can actually block the flow of air through one side of the nose. On rare occasions, it can deviate in both directions, causing symptoms of stuffiness on both sides of the nose.

TABLE 8-3
Commonly Prescribed Medications That Can
Cause Systemic Rhinitis Medicamentosa*

Medication (Brand Name)	NASAL SYMPTOM(S) PRODUCED			
	Congestion	Runny Nose	Bleeding	Dry Nose
Accutane				•
Aldomet	•			
Ansaid			•	
BuSpar	•		•	
Capoten		•		
Cardizem	•		•	
Catapres				•
Cipro			•	
Clinoril			•	
Combipres				•
Compazine	•		•	
Corgard	•			
Demulen		•		
Desyrel	•			
Dramamine				•
Emcyt		•		
Enovid		•		
Feldene			•	
Indocin			•	
Intal	•		•	
Klonopin		•		
Lortab ASA		•		
Lozol		•		
Marax				•
Minipress	•		•	
Moduretic	•			
Motrin		•	•	
Nicorette			•	
Normozide		•		
Norzine				•
Orudis			•	

Medication (Brand Name)	Congestion	Runny Nose	Bleeding	Dry Nose
Procardia	•			
Proventil	•		•	
Prozac	•		•	
Reserpine	•			
Soma		•		
Tegison				•
Timoptic	•			
Torecan				•
Trental	•		•	
Vasotec		•		
Voltaren			•	
Xanax	•			
Zestril	•			

* SOURCE: Side-Effects and Interactions, PDR, 1990, and American Druggist, February, 1990

Cleft Palate. The palate is the roof of your mouth. When it does not develop properly, it leaves a large opening in the roof of the mouth. This causes the nose and the mouth to connect abnormally, and results in many different problems for someone so affected.

Choanal Atresia (Bilateral). The term *choanal* (funnel) refers to the shape of each side of the nose from the outside toward the throat. The term *atresia* (no hole) refers to the lack of an opening at the end of this funnel. Someone with bilateral choanal atresia has no opening into the throat for either of the nasal passageways, and no air can pass through the nose to the lungs. Choanal Atresia is a life-threatening situation for an infant.

Pharyngeal Stenosis. This is a very uncommon disorder in which the pharynx, located at the back of the nose and the top of the throat, is abnormally narrowed. Just as in a pinched pipe, such narrowing does not permit normal flow of air or fluid through the nose.

Benign Tumors. There are a variety of abnormal but not cancerous (benign) growths that can occur in the nasal passageways. These may block the flow of air through the nose on the side in which they occur. Nasal Polyps, balloon like swellings of the lining of the nose, are the most common of these.

Anatomic Causes of a Nonallergic Runny Nose

If you or your child suffer from a chronic runny nose, you may have one of the five disorders listed below. Surgical correction of each is frequently required.

Adenoid hypertrophy. Lymphoid tissue (immune protection cells) line the back of the throat and extend up, behind the nose. When bacteria, viruses, or other agents stimulate the cells of this tissue, the cells multiply, and the amount of tissue increases significantly (hypertrophy). This increase can be large enough to interfere with the passage of air through the nose.

Choanal Atresia (Unilateral). While bilateral choanal atresia affects both sides of the nose, people with unilateral choanal atresia have one nasal passageway that is incompletely formed and fails to connect with the back of the throat. For them, nasal congestion is not a major symptom, as you might think it would be, because people with this abnormality have had it since birth. To them it is "normal" to breathe through only one side of the nose, the blockage of the other side goes unnoticed.

CSF Rhinorrhea. Cerebrospinal fluid (CSF) is the fluid that circulates in and around the brain and spinal column. Rarely, following certain infections and injuries, the CSF can actually leak into the nasal cavity. When it does it usually runs out the front of the nose, thus causing a "runny nose." Hence the term CSF rhinorrhea. It is not unusual for someone with this disorder to be able to produce a runny nose simply by looking down and leaning over.

Foreign Bodies. Anything that can fit into the nose may someday be found in a nose. Children often place objects in the nose, and may push them in too far to get them out. If you discover that your child has done this, the object should be removed by a doctor right away. If an object put into the nose stays there a while, it will cause an inflammation and perhaps an infection of the lining of the nose where it is lodged. This will cause an oozing of fluid from the lining of the nose, and that will cause a runny nose from the side involved. A foul odor arising from the nose is also frequently present.

Tumors (Cancer). Cancerous tumors can and do occur in the nose and, when they cause symptoms, a runny nose is common. Such tumors are rare in children.

"If it's not a cold, it must be an allergy. Right?" Now, you know the answer.

QUESTIONS AND ANSWERS

1. I've been using an over-the-counter nasal decongestant spray every day for two years. Every time I try to stop, my nose becomes so stuffy that I can't breathe. How can I get off of this spray?

The first thing you need to do is talk to your doctor about this. The quickest and easiest way for you to break the habit of nasal sprays is by the combined use of a decongestant taken by mouth, nasal corticosteroid sprays, and a short course of corticosteroids taken by mouth. These agents combine to reduce the inflammation and swelling associated with chronic abuse of over-the-counter nasal decongestant sprays and to prevent the mechanism of rebound responsible for the habit. This combination should allow you to discontinue your nasal spray without sleepless nights within five days. Depending upon how long you have been using decongestant nasal sprays, you may need to take the corticosteroid nasal spray for one to three months; but don't worry, you won't get hooked on it.

2. My daughter has a deviated septum, but her doctor said that it did not need to be fixed. Is that OK?
Most people have some slight deviation of their nasal septum, not enough to cause symptoms. If your daughter's deviated septum is not causing nasal problems—stuffiness, bleeding, contributing to recurring sinus infections—then it is nothing more than something a physician will observe, and perhaps comment upon, when he looks into her nose.

3. What is Sampter's syndrome? My doctor said that I have it, but I didn't quite understand what she meant.
A person has Sampter's syndrome when he or she has a combination of medical problems: bronchial asthma, chronic sinusitis, nasal polyps, and a very abnormal, allergic-like reaction to aspirin and medications similar in action to aspirin. This reaction to aspirin may include nasal congestion, severe asthma, generalized urticaria (hives), allergic shock, and even death. These people, like anyone who experiences an abnormal reaction to a medication, should completely avoid that and similar medications. If you have this problem, discuss with your doctor which medications you should completely avoid.

4. How can you tell whether your runny nose is nasal mucus or cerebrospinal fluid?
First of all, frequently the runny nose caused by leaking cerebrospinal fluid greatly worsens when you bend over to pick up something: regular runny noses do not. Second, cerebrospinal fluid contains a significant amount of sugar, which can be detected by a simple laboratory test. Regular nasal mucus does not contain sugar. Third, very sophisticated X-ray type tests can confirm a cerebrospinal fluid leak and pinpoint its location.

PART FOUR

Getting to Know
Your Nose

CHAPTER 9

WHAT TYPE OF NOSE PROBLEM DO YOU HAVE?

Now it's time for you to begin to pinpoint the type(s) of rhinitis you have. This is your chapter. I'll provide the questions, you provide the answers. The questions are divided into sections for each type of rhinitis and are designed to help you easily identify the type(s) of rhinitis you have. Completing the questionnaire will help you better understand your symptoms as well as form the basis for understanding the treatment options available to you, which will be discussed in chapters 10-18.

NOTE: This questionnaire is intended to be used in cooperation with your physician. The final determination of the type(s) of rhinitis troubling you will be up to your doctor.

Instructions: Either indicate by a check mark or write in the correct response to the following questions.

WHICH OF THE FOLLOWING NASAL SYMPTOMS DO YOU TYPICALLY HAVE?

Stuffy nose	__	Runny nose	__
Postnasal drainage	__	·Sneezing	__
Nose bleeding	__	Dry nose	__
Itchy nose	__	Loss of sense of smell	__
Itchy roof of the mouth	__	Itchy throat	__
		Itchy deep inside ears	__

How Long Have You Had Nose Problems?

For how many months or years have you been having nasal symptoms typical of those you currently are experiencing? (Fill in the total amount of time, not just how long you've had trouble this year or season.)

_____

In General, Are Your Symptoms Getting Better, Worse, Or Are They Unchanged Since They Began?

Better_____ Worse_____ Unchanged_____

If Your Symptoms Are Changing, Do You Know Any Reason(s) For The Change?
Are any external factors (a move, change of jobs, taking medications, etc.) coincident with the change?

_____

_____

How Severe Are Your Symptoms?

Mild_____
Mild symptoms would be those that you notice, but that do not cause you any significant discomfort.

Moderate_____
Moderate symptoms are those that cause you discomfort and for which you have to take medication intermittently.

Severe_____
Severe symptoms are those that cause you significant discomfort and for which you require daily or near-daily medication in order to obtain relief.

What Are The Times(s) Of Day When Your Symptoms Most Often Occur?

In the morning when I first awaken   _____
Around noon   _____
In the late afternoon   _____
In the evening before I go to bed   _____
During the night, while I try to sleep   _____
My symptoms seem to last all day, but they don't
  bother me at night   _____
My symptoms seem to occur during the night,
  but not during the day   _____
My symptoms are present all the time   _____

What Is The Time of Week When Your Symptoms Most Often Occur?

If there is (are) any day(s) of the week on which your symptoms are increased, please list it (them) here:

If you suspect a reason (at work, on weekends, at grandmother's, etc.), please say so here:

Which Month(s) of the Year Do Your Symptoms Occur?

January	_____	July	_____
February	_____	August	_____
March	_____	September	_____
April	_____	October	_____
May	_____	November	_____
June	_____	December	_____

Do You Have Any Other Symptoms That Seem To Occur With Or Around The Time Of Your Nasal Symptoms?

Headache	___	Dizziness	___
Watery eyes	___	Bronchitis	___
Hoarseness	___	Mouth breathing	___
Sinusitis	___	Snoring	___
Nasal speech	___	Red eyes	___
Sleeping problems	___	Ear infections	___
Decrease or loss of		Loss of taste	___
sense of smell	___	Pneumonia	___
Sore throat	___	Fatigue	___
Itchy eyes	___	Nose bleeding	___

Any others?

Do Your Nasal Symptoms Interfere With Your Life?

My symptoms interfere with things I want to do, such as the following:

My symptoms interfere with things I must do, such as the following:

THE RHINITIS SYNDROMES

I. Allergic Nasal Syndromes
A. Seasonal Allergic Rhinitis
My symptoms occur *only* during pollen season:
YES_____ NO_____

If *YES*, please check the season(s) during which your symptoms occur:

Early spring	____	Late spring	____
Summer	____	Fall	____
Winter	____		

B. Perennial Allergic Rhinitis

My symptoms can occur any time of the year, they are not limited to just one pollen season.

YES____ NO____

If *YES*, please indicate which of the following seem to trigger your symptoms:

Dusting, sweeping, cleaning, vacuuming   ____
Raking leaves, musty smells, compost piles, fertilizer   ____
Dogs   ____
Cats   ____
Birds   ____
Feather pillows   ____
Horses   ____
Tree pollen   ____
Freshly cut grass during the late spring and early summer ____
During the fall (weed pollen season)   ____
Certain foods that I eat   ____

If you checked the previous blank, please indicate which foods you suspect as causes of your nasal symptoms:

_____

_____

Other allergy triggers? List them here:

_____

_____

C. Occupational Allergic Rhinitis

Where do you work?_____

Type of business? _____

Briefly describe your job:_____

_____

Are you exposed at work to any agent that is known to cause work-associated allergies?

YES_____ NO_____

If *YES*, then list the names of these agents:

_____

Do your symptoms seem worse when you are at work?

YES_____ NO_____

Do you suspect any specific cause?

YES_____ NO_____

If *YES*, please list the agents that you suspect as causes of your symptoms:

_____

How many people work in the same area as you?_____

Do any of them have a problem similar to yours:

YES_____ NO_____

If *YES*, how many?_____

Indicate whether your symptoms are better, worse, or unchanged
in relation to:

Work Time	Better	Worse	Unchanged
Early in the work week	_____	_____	_____
End of work week	_____	_____	_____
Weekends or when not working	_____	_____	_____
Vacations/holidays	_____	_____	_____

II. NonAllergic Nasal Syndromes

These are listed in the order in which they appear in chapter 8.

A. Nonanatomic Rhinitis

1. Atrophic Rhinitis
My main nose symptom is a dry nose ☐
I have lots of crusts in my nose ☐
There seems to always be a foul smell in my nose ☐

2. Cold Air Rhinitis
Does being outside in cold air trigger or worsen your nasal symptoms?
YES_____ NO_____

3. Eosinophilic Rhinitis
I have asthma ☐
I react abnormally to aspirin ☐
I have nasal polyps ☐
I have chronic or repeated sinus infections ☐

4. Hormone/Endocrine Rhinitis
Indicate if any of the following apply to you:
I have a low-functioning thyroid gland ☐
I am taking birth-control pills ☐
I am taking estrogen pills ☐
When I am pregnant, my nose symptoms worsen ☐
My nose symptoms worsen in relation to ☐
  my menstrual cycle:
During my period ☐
Just before my period ☐
Just after my period ☐
In the middle of my monthly cycle ☐

5. Immunologic Rhinitis
As discussed in chapter 8, the absence of any of the immune protective factors causes an increased susceptibility to infections. The only way you would know if you have this problem is for your physician to have al-

ready made this diagnosis. If you do have an immune deficiency disorder, please list its name:

6. *Infectious Rhinitis*
Do you seem to have a cold almost all the time?
YES____ NO____

How many colds do you get per year?

Are you exposed to people who seem to get several colds per year?
YES____ NO____

Have you had any of the following in the past two years?

Sinusitis	____	Infected Ears	____
Bronchitis	____	Pneumonia	____

7. *Irritant Rhinitis*
a) Chemicals in the air
Are your symptoms caused or worsened by exposure to any of the following?

Chemicals	____	Cleaning agents	____
Cologne	____	Cooking odors	____
Detergents	____	Deodorants	____
Hair spray	____	Industrial fumes	____
Insecticides	____	Newsprint	____
Paint fumes	____	Perfume	____
Smoke	____	Hair solutions	____

Other(s): _____

b) Dusts
If your symptoms are caused or worsened by exposure to dust particles, what type of dust

(house, yard, barn, etc.) seems to trigger symptoms?

_____

_____

c) Smokes
Do any of the following smokes cause or worsen your nasal symptoms?

Cigarette	____	Pipe	____
Campfire	____	Trash burning	____
Cigar	____		

Other smokes:_____

d) Powders
   Do any of the following cause or worsen your nasal symptoms?
   Body powder   ____
   Detergent powder   ____
   Other powders   ____

e) Cosmetics
   Do any of the following cause or worsen your nose symptoms?

Perfumes	____	Colognes	____
Lotions	____	Aftershave	____
Creams	____	Makeup	____
Powder	____	Foundation	____

   Other: _____

f) Chemicals
   Do any of the following cause or worsen your nose symptoms?

Automobile exhuasts	____	Insecticides	____
Pollution	____	Gasoline	____
Paint	____		

g) Others
  If there are any other irritating substances that you
  suspect are either causing or worsening your
  symptoms, please list them here: _____
  _____

8   *Primary Nasal Mastocytosis*
  There are no specific questions to ask that would help
  focus in on this type on nose problem, since its
  diagnosis will depend on your physical examination
  and additional tests your doctor may order. See page
  101 for a discussion of this form of rhinitis.

9. *Reflex Rhinitis*
  Do you have nose symptoms in the following
  situations:
  Are exposed to bright lights   _____
  Lie on your side   _____
  Get cold   _____
  Are stressed (anxious,
      afraid, angry, or worried)   _____
  Exercise   _____
  Eating or just after eating   _____

10. *Rhinitis Medicamentosa*
  a) Local
  Are you using or have you recently been using nasal
  decongestant sprays or drops?
              YES____ NO____
  If *Yes*, which spray(s) have you used?
  Afrin   _____
  Dristan   _____
  Neosynephrine   _____
  Other: _____
  How many times in 24 hours do you usually use
  these?_____
  b) Systemic
  Are you taking any medications for blood pressure, heart,
  stomach, stress, or skin or other medical problems?

YES____ NO____
If *YES*, please check the ones you use:

Medication Function	Brand Name
Antiacne	Accutane
Antianxiety	BuSpar
	Limbitrol
Anticonvulsant	Klonopin
Antidepressants	Adalat
	Etrafon
	Ludiomil
Antinausea	Dramamine
	Norzine
	Torecan
Antipsychotics	Navane
	Serentil
Antiviral	Retrovir
Blood Pressure Control	Azactam
	Capoten
	Cardizem
	Catapres
	Combipres
	Esimil
	Harmonyl
	Hydropres
	Lozol
	Normozide
	Vasotec
Bronchodilator	Marax
Circulatory	Disopyramide phosphate
	Trental
Chemotherapy	Emcyt
	Intron A
	Sandostatin
Cough Suppressant	Tessalon
Hormones Supplement	Danocrine
	Enovid

Medication Function	Brand Name
Muscle Relaxants	Lioresal
	Soma
Pain Reliever	Lortab ASA
	Motrin
Psoriasis Control	Tegison

Other medications: _____

_____

_____

11. Vasomotor Rhinitis
    Your doctor will have to help you here, because you
    can have this problem only if you do not have any of
    the above types of nasal problems.

B. Anatomic

Any of the following types of anatomic problems could
contribute to or cause your symptoms. Your doctor will
be able to tell you whether or not any of the following
apply to you. Indicate by a check mark those identified by
your doctor during your physical examination.

1. Congestive Syndromes
(Primary Symptom = Stuffy Nose)
Deviated nasal septum
Cleft palate   ___
Choanal atresia (both sides)   ___
Pharyngeal stenosis   ___
Benign tumors   ___
                                                ___

2. Rhinorrhea Syndromes
(Primary Symptom = Runny Nose)
Adenoid enlargement
Choanal atresia (one side)   ___
CSF rhinorrhea   ___
Foreign body   ___
Cancer   ___
                                                ___

Now That You've Answered All Of These Questions, What Should You Do?

First of all, if you are unsure about any question, make a note to discuss it with your doctor.
List in the space below each of the different types of rhinitis under which you indicated you had symptoms: _____

_____

_____

_____

_____

_____

You should now have a good idea of the different types of rhinitis that could be causing your nasal symptoms. If you've listed more than one cause, it should be clear that your symptoms may at one time be due to one form of rhinitis, while at another time they may be due to another form of rhinitis.

The Next Step: See Your Doctor

I suggest that you take this book, or a copy of these pages of questions, to your doctor. After reviewing them, chances are your doctor will want to ask some additional questions and then examine you to be sure there are no anatomic problems contributing to your rhinitis. Occasionally, X-rays may be needed.

Consultation with a specialist in allergy may be needed if allergy triggers are playing a role in causing your symptoms.

Once your evaluation has been completed, your doctor can sit down with you and discuss what can be done to help you feel better. The various strategies that your doctor might employ in helping you are detailed in chapters 10-18.

QUESTIONS AND ANSWERS

1. I'm taking two of the blood pressure pills listed in the questionnaire, and I am experiencing nasal symptoms. What should I do?

Call your doctor and discuss this. As discussed in chapter 8, it is possible to suffer nasal symptoms as a side effect of certain medications; however, only a small percentage of people who take these medications experience nasal side effects. Your doctor can help you determine whether or not they are actually playing a role in causing your symptoms.

Important: Do not under any circumstances change or stop any current medication regimen without consulting your doctor.

2. My symptoms did not begin until I was twenty-six years old. I thought that if you were allergic, you were born that way.

You are, but what you are born with is the ability to become allergic at some point in your life, provided you are exposed to the things to which you have inherited the ability to react allergically. Just when, if ever, your body becomes allergic and you begin getting nasal symptoms will vary considerably.

3. My brother-in-law has always been susceptible to colds, but in adulthood he's begun having them even more often, along with repeated sinus infections. His doctor says that he doesn't make IgA antibodies. Where does this diagnosis fit into a differential diagnosis?

The lack of ability to produce IgA, an antibody that is present in nasal and other body fluids, is an immune deficiency disease. In fact, it is the most common immune deficiency disease, occurring in 1 in every 500 people. The absence of IgA increases one's susceptability to infection. IgA deficiency is an example of a nonallergic cause for rhinitis.

CHAPTER 10

AVOIDANCE: THE BEST OF ALL TREATMENTS

"AN OUNCE OF PREVENTION is worth a pound of cure," observed Benjamin Franklin. Nowhere in medicine are these words more true than in the treatment of allergic, or twitchy, noses.

The single most important aspect of the treatment of your chronic rhinitis is *avoidance*: of pollens, dust, dust mites, mold spores, dogs, cats, smoke, chemical agents, aerosols, or whatever else aggravates your nasal symptoms. It is ironic that although avoidance measures are the single most effective, least expensive, and least complicated of treatment options, they are also the least heeded. It is as if we would take a pill, squirt a spray, get an injection, or all three rather than inconvenience ourselves with avoidance measures—even though avoidance measures work wonderfully well.

This chapter will describe how to avoid effectively the more common agents causing or triggering chronic rhinitis.

AVOIDING HOUSE DUST

House dust (chapter 6) is the sum of your environmental accumulations. It is, so to speak, the crumbs on the floor of your cave. It is a mixture of dried food particles, outside dust, pollen particles, mold spores, various fibers, insect parts and droppings, pesticides, and, from indoor pets, hair, shed skin cells, saliva, and urine. It's not "one thing," like oak pollen, or cigarette smoke. Worse, it's everywhere you look, feel, walk, sit, stand, lie and breathe—unless you control it.

If your nose reacts to house dust, the following are suggestions that will go a long way toward helping you reduce your house dust exposure:

1. Focus your efforts on your bedroom. It is most important to have at least one room in which dust is optimally controlled. For most of us, this is the bedroom, because it is the room in the home where we spend most of our at-home hours.

2. Know your level of exposure. Begin your control of house dust by establishing the degree of your dust exposure in the bedroom. This can be done by completing the checklist in table 10-1.

TABLE 10-1
House Dust Exposure Check List

Check the items that apply to your bedroom. The more items you check, the greater is your exposure to house dust.

☐ Carpet
☐ Fabric upholstered furniture
☐ Drapes or Curtains
☐ Venetian blinds
☐ Louvered blinds of any type
☐ Pictures/posters on wall
☐ Cloth headboard on bed
☐ Canopy over bed
☐ Skirt around bed
☐ Fuzzy blankets
☐ Stuffed toys
☐ No vinyl encasements for pillow, mattress, or springs
☐ Book shelves, books
☐ Cabinets
☐ Closet in the room

☐ Closet full of shoes, clothes
☐ Many boxes in closet
☐ No special filter on central air system or in room
☐ Room is damp dusted and/or mopped less than once/wk
☐ Room is cleaned/vacuumed less than once/wk
☐ I clean/vacuum my room myself

3. Clear the room. Remove *everything* from the room, its closets, cabinets, and shelves: furniture, drapes, curtains, books, pictures, knickknacks, mattress, springs, clothes, shoes, and carpet. Noncarpeted floors and bare windows are best. Washable cotton curtains or those made of plastic are easy to clean.

4. Clean the room thoroughly, ceiling to floor. Damp dust rather than dry dust, and mop rather than sweep. Don't forget the closet: it's a very dusty place.

5. Clean the bed and other furniture in another area outside is best.

6. Return to your room only those pieces of furniture that are essential. In deciding which pieces to return, keep in mind that when dust-proofing a room, "less is best." A bed, a table, a chair, a dresser almost always serve the room's purpose. Wood, plastic, metal, or vinyl furniture is preferred, as these surfaces are easily maintained.

7. Encase pillows, mattress, and springs in air-tight, vinyl encasements available in most department stores.

8. Store only frequently-used clothing in your bedroom closet. Place this clothing in air-tight, zipper-sealed, vinyl clothes-bags.

9. Close the air conditioning vent into the room.

10. Have someone else clean the room, if possible. It is

best for the dust-allergic person not to be the one to clean the room. You should be away from the room for four or more hours after its cleaning. If this is not possible, and you are the one cleaning the room, wear a mask while cleaning. Simple, inexpensive dust masks (the 3M Dust and Pollen Filter Mask is an example) can be purchased in drugstores. If these are not sufficient, more sophisticated masks can be ordered from several suppliers (appendix 3).

11. Don't use your bedroom as a storeroom. It is important that your dust-free room not be used to store things. That includes books, clothing, shoes, toys, magazines. The more things in a room, the more dust will accumulate.

12. Wash bedding weekly.

13. Establish a routine for regular cleaning of the room. Damp mopping and dusting daily will slow the reaccumulation of dust, but dust will reaccumulate. A more thorough cleaning (walls, ceiling, window shades or blinds, closet) once weekly is essential to maintain good dust control.

14. Install an air filter. There are several types of filters that can effectively clear the air in your home of pollen, dust, mold spores, and animal allergens. They work on one of two general concepts:

• Mechanical Filtration. Particles are removed by this filter because their size prevents them from traversing the system. The efficiency of systems using this mode of clearance can be as high as 99.99 percent when a high efficiency particulate accumulator (HEPA) system is used.

• Electrostatic Filtration. Particles are removed by first being given a negative electrical charge. Then they are attracted to and trapped on wires with a positive electrical charge. Although highly effective when first installed, these filters quickly lose their effectiveness because of the accumulation of particles on the wire components. People who use these systems successfully clean them weekly.

A listing of some manufacturers from whom home filters can be purchased is provided in appendix IV

15. If you purchase a stand-alone filter system for a single room instead of one for your central system, one with a HEPA filter is best. However, be sure you get a large enough system that turns the air in the room many times each hour. The emphasis here is on the term *large*. Tabletop filters are not adequate to filter the air in your entire room. Most bedrooms require a unit about the size of an end table.

AVOIDING HOUSE DUST MITES

There are seven basic steps to take in reducing your exposure to house dust mites:

1. Put vinyl encasements around your pillow, mattress, and springs.
2. Hot water wash your bedding once a week.
3. Remove carpet from the bedroom. This is very important, as the carpet is the major nest for the house dust mite.
4. Install an air filtration system on your central system, your window air conditioner, or as a stand alone unit in your bedroom (Appendix IV).
5. Double-bag you vacuum cleaner.
6. Install a filter on the outlet port of your vacuum cleaner Appendix III).
7. Wear a mask when vacuuming.

The most important of these is the removal of carpet from the bedroom. It is in the carpet where the house mites most often make their homes—it's their nest. While removing bedroom carpet is a step many are reluctant to take, it is *the best way* to reduce mites. Many studies show the importance of carpet removal in limiting both your exposure to mites and the symptoms they cause. These same studies also suggest that if the carpet is not removed, your symptoms are likely to continue.

If removing your carpet is simply not an option, **Acarosan powder** can help. As discussed in chapter 6, it is the droppings, not the mites themselves, to which mite-allergic people react. Acarosan powder kills house mites and clumps them together with their droppings, making removal by vacuuming effective. This product is expensive and requires application every two to three months, but it is very effective.

If you are allergic to several agents—pollens, mold spores, dogs or cats, *and* house mites for example—it is still best to remove the carpet. Acarosan will not help control the accumulation of pollen, dog or cat particles, or mold spores. Acarosan powder is available from your pharmacist without a prescription. A little kit for testing your dust for mites is also available so you can monitor how well your mite reduction efforts are working.

AVOIDING MOLD SPORES

The three Ds of avoiding mold spores are darkness, dampness, and drafts: molds abound in environments of low or no light, increased humidity, and the absence of ventilation or drafts. Begin your mold avoidance program as you did your dust program: by first determining your level and sites of exposure to mold spores. Table 10-2 should help.

TABLE 10-2
Mold Spore Exposure Checklist

Check the conditions that apply to you. The more checks, the greater is your exposure to mold spores.

Outside your home:
- ☐ Very shady yard, little direct light
- ☐ Vegetation is dense
- ☐ Compost pile present
- ☐ Pine straw accumulations
- ☐ Leaf accumulations
- ☐ Cut grass accumulations
- ☐ Standing water is a problem in spots
- ☐ It smells moldy in your yard
- ☐ You have a greenhouse
- ☐ You have a barn and/or stables
- ☐ You have a poolhouse

☐ You have an awning
☐ You have a kennel
☐ There is a crawl space under your house
☐ There is standing water around your house

Inside your home:
☐ You have a basement
☐ Basement is poorly, infrequently lighted
☐ Basement is poorly ventilated
☐ Basement smells moldy sometimes
☐ Basement "sweats"
☐ Bathroom walls are moldy
☐ Shower or tub walls, doors, or curtains are moldy
☐ Sink/area under sink is moldy
☐ Tiling/area around toilet is moldy
☐ Bathroom carpet is frequently moist
☐ Bathroom is poorly ventilated
☐ Kitchen sink/under sink is moist or moldy
☐ Garbage area/garbage pail smells moldy
☐ Area around/under refrigerator is moldy
☐ Some food inside refrigerator is moldy
☐ Bookcases/books are moldy
☐ Tape cases/tapes are moldy
☐ Pet litter boxes are moldy
☐ Pet sleeping area is moldy
☐ The walls in your house are moldy
☐ Water sometimes leaks into your home

In addition, the following conditions promote mold growth in your home: Walls without mold-retarding paint, fruits and vegetables whether in the open or inside the refrigerator, bread, old books, old boxes, storage rooms, shower stall, shower doors or curtains, clothes hampers, pet food, room humidifiers, central heat humidifiers, central air conditioning system, ducts of central air conditioning system, and Christmas trees.

The Three Ds

Keep the three Ds in mind as you review the following actions you might take to reduce your exposure to outdoor mold spores:

Dampness

1. Avoid, if and when possible, places where the humidity is high: basements, camps on the lake, clothes hampers, greenhouses, stables, and barns.

2. Dampness in the home caused by water leakage is a prime source of mold-spore accumulation. If your home seems continually damp, look for possible sources of leakage and correct them.

3. Carpeting, including padding, that has been extensively wetted and wood that has rotted as a result of water leakage are best replaced.

4. Although indoor plants cause few mold problems, the containers in which these plants are housed can be a problem because they are frequently wet from the water for the plant. Sometimes, plants may even rest in containers of water.

5. Keeping your windows sealed as tightly as possible will help. In older homes, weather stripping or plastic tape may be needed. In newer homes, the windows generally seal properly.

6. Dehumidifiers are infrequently helpful. Your resources will be better spent on improved sealing of windows and doors.

Darkness

1. A light in a basement may help decrease mold growth. Connected to a timer, it should be easy to light this space several hours each day.

2. Consider a small light in closets, one that comes on when you turn on the room light.

3. Consider the addition of windows to any dark room.

Absence of Ventilation (Drafts)

1. Ventilate closed rooms: open doors, install fans.

2. Check your ventilation system to be sure that it is working optimally.

3. If you are using a basement as part of your living area, its ventilation should be included in that of the other parts of your home.

4. Install a small fan in an area that is poorly ventilated and turn it on regularly.

AVOIDING POLLENS

Pollen is everywhere, and it flourishes where most people live. There are exceptions, such as at the polar caps and at very high altitudes, but these are sufficiently inaccessible to most of us to be, essentially, irrelevant.

The following are general guidelines that can reduce both your exposure to the ubiquitous pollens and the symptoms that result from that exposure:

1. Staying inside with closed doors and windows is the best way to reduce your exposure to pollens during your particular pollen season(s).

2. Window fans and attic fans are infamous for drawing pollens into homes. Any type of fan can stir up mite particles, mold spores, animal danders, and pollens already within your home. In general, if you are allergic to a variety of inhaled indoor and outdoor allergens, it is best not to use fans in your home.

4. Putting the car air conditioner on "recirculate" while driving will help reduce pollen exposure.

5. Obviously, outdoor activities and yard work during your pollen season(s) can worsen your symptoms. If you are grass- or tree-pollen allergic, try to have someone else tend your yard during the weed, grass, and tree pollen seasons.

5. Don't hang clothes or bedding outside to dry, as they become pollen catchers.

7. A good filter on your central air/heat system or a

standalone filtering unit in your bedroom can be very helpful. Remember, though, filters filter. Since these filter systems work effectively only as long as they are kept clean, wash them weekly during your allergy season(s).

8. It is best if you are not the one to hose down, blow, or sweep the yellow pollen off of your driveway, porch or patio.

9. Get out of town—way out of town—during your season(s). If possible, plan your vacation and go to an area not filled with the pollen(s) to which you are allergic. If only we could escape for an entire season!

Getting away during a pollen season does work for some people, especially people who are very reactive to only a single pollen such as ragweed. They can go where the counts are generally very low, places like Florida, the big island of Hawaii, Alaska, eastern Canada, the Virgin Islands, or even Bermuda. If you live in south central Texas and happen to be very reactive only to mountain cedar pollen, you can go almost anywhere else and get relief during your season.

Unfortunately, most people with chronic allergic rhinitis are reactive to many different allergens: pollens, dusts, mites, and molds. So, even though they might vacation away from ragweed, they are likely to discover that their vacation paradise has grass or tree pollens, or mites and mold spores in abundance—that they have even worse allergies on vacation than they do at home.

Before you rush off someplace, be sure you're not going from the frying pan into the fire. Talk to your allergist. Don't go to Florida to avoid the high ragweed counts of northern Virginia, only to run into tree pollen to which you are also allergic. Don't take the family to sunny California, thinking it safely away from New Jersey in September, only to discover that the ragweed pollen in California, like that in New Jersey, is raging at that time of year.

AVOIDING CAT ALLERGENS

Removing the pet from the interior of the home of the cat allergic person is clearly the most effective way to manage an allergy to cats. Symptoms may not improve significantly for some two months following the pet's removal, however.

Again, special central system filters can prove helpful to a cat-allergic person. As discussed in chapter 6, cat allergen, Fel d 1, is easily airborne and has a long "hang" time. Its time aloft, however, may be long enough to permit an air conditioning unit to capture and filter it.

Outdoor cats are not a major problem, so long as the allergic person does not have close contact with them. However, if a highly cat-allergic person elects to go outside, hold the cat in his or her lap, and pet and hug the cat, significant symptoms can result. In addition, the cat "comes in" on the clothes.

Carpet Removal, Steam Cleaning, Vacuuming

The effectiveness of carpet removal, steam cleaning, and vacuuming for getting rid of cat allergen cannot be recommended. You can reduce the allergy-causing ability of cat allergen in your home by spraying a tannic acid solution (Allergen Inhibitor Solution) into your carpet and furniture on a regular basis. To avoid staining and color changes, follow the direction of the manufacturer closely.

To date, the most effective measure one can take in reducing exposure to cat allergen is to remove the cat from the home. If you are not willing to do this, you may need to resign yourself to a life of symptoms, pills, sprays, and/or shots. If you aren't going to get the cat out of the house, then at least give your little feline friend a bath, regularly. Your veterinarian can provide directions for bathing your cat. Doing this weekly will help reduce your exposure to cat allergen.

AVOIDING DOG ALLERGEN

Like cat allergens, dog allergens are best dealt with either by not having a dog or by keeping it 100 percent outside. If there is a question regarding the importance of the dog allergen, then a trial removal from the home for 4 to 6 weeks might be considered. To be meaningful, such a trial removal should be accompanied by a thorough cleaning of the area(s) in which the dog has lived, shortly after the dog's departure.

AVOIDING SMOKE

The presence of a smoker in the home will sabotage the best of all possible treatment programs for rhinitis.
If you have a chronic rhinitis problem, don't smoke. If someone else in your family or home suffers from it, don't smoke. Smoking may be the reason why rhinitis symptoms are continuing in spite of an otherwise intelligent treatment program. Your smoke also may be the reason why your child or spouse gets so many colds, bronchitis, and ear infections or has so much trouble with asthma.

If you smoke, quit. It's bad for your nose and lungs, and the noses and lungs of everyone else who lives with you.

QUESTIONS AND ANSWERS

1. What is the most effective agent for decreasing mold spores?
While aerosol sprays help counter the smell of mold in the air, only soaking solutions, such as Clorox, can combat mold growth.

2. Someone told me that my newspaper would not burn my nose and eyes or make them run if I cooked it first. Is that right?
Some people find that baking a newspaper before they read

it eliminates the odors of newsprint enough so they can read it without sneezing or suffering from a burning or runny nose. However, most people who are bothered by newsprint find that if someone else first simply lays the paper out and slowly turns each page, from front to rear, they can then read it without symptoms. Try this first. However, if this doesn't work, bake it at 200 degrees F, but keep careful watch during this process to avoid a fire.

3. You focused on the bedroom for the first part of this chapter What about the rest of the house?

You can apply the ideas presented in this chapter to any room of your home, but first apply them to your bedroom. Once you have done everything that can be done in your bedroom, the next room to focus on would be the room where you spend the next most time. For me, this would be the room where I write. For someone else, this might be a family room, a workshop, the living room, or the kitchen.

4. Why should I give up smoking just because my kid has a nose problem?

If your child has a frequent or persistent nasal problem, exposure to tobacco smoke will aggravate the situation. This heightens your child's symptoms as well as their frequency and the likelihood of complications such as sinusitis, otitis, bronchitis, and pneumonia. The result is an increase in the number and frequency of medications your child will require, of visits to the doctor, of school absenteeism, and an increase in the overall cost of your child's medical care.

PART FIVE

Taking Care of Your Nose

CHAPTER 11

THE ANTIHISTAMINES

THE WORD *antihistamine* is a combination of terms: *anti*, meaning against, and *histamine*, a naturally-occurring bodily chemical that regulates a variety of bodily activities and is a chemical mediator (chapter 3) of both allergic and nonallergic forms of chronic rhinitis.

Histamine is present in the mast cells (chapter 3) of the lining of your nose. Not only does it participate in normal nasal function, during allergic reactions it is released in abundance into the surrounding tissue where it becomes the primary mediator of common nasal symptoms: runny nose, sneezing, itchy nose, postnasal drainage, and stuffy nose.

Histamine exerts its effect on the tissues of the nose through special structures on those tissues called *histamine receptors.* If there is no receptor for histamine, it cannot act on your tissues. No action on tissues, no symptoms. This fact becomes important in discussing how certain drugs act to counter the effects of histamine.

Humans have three different types of histamine receptors: H1, H2, and H3 receptors. These receptors are located on most tissues in our bodies. Different tissue effects are produced through histamine's action on each of these receptors. It is through the H1 receptors that histamine exerts its effect on our noses. The actions that result from histamine acting with H2 or H3 receptors are currently not believed to play an important role in causing nasal symptoms.

Table 11-1 shows some of the changes caused by histamine when it acts on H1 receptors.

TABLE 11-1
Nasal Symptoms Caused by Histamine Acting on Tissue H1 Receptors

Symptom	Histamine Action on H1 Receptor
Nasal congestion	Dilation of blood vessels, leaking of plasma from blood vessels into surrounding tissue
Sneezing	Reflex stimulation
Itching of nose	Reflex stimulation

How Antihistamines Work

Antihistamines work against (anti = against) histamine by competing with it for H1 receptors. Antihistamines as a group are commonly called H1 antagonists, because they impede the H1-receptor effects of histamine.

H I receptors can act with only one agent at a time; thus, when they are acting with antihistamines, they cannot act with histamine. If histamine can't act with the H1 receptor, it can't cause any changes in your nose. And, if there are no nasal changes, you suffer no symptoms.

The Classes of Antihistamines

Antihistamines have been around for almost 50 years. You know them as medications to be taken when you need relief from the following:
* Runny nose
* Sneezing
* Postnasal drip
* Itchy nose, throat, roof of the mouth, or ears

* Red, watery, itchy eyes commonly associated with
  allergic nasal symptoms

What you probably don't know is that there are eight classes of antihistamines (table 11-2), each important for a different reason.

TABLE 11-2
The Eight Classes of Antihistamines

Class	Chemical Name	Generic Name	Manufacturer's Name or Common Name
I	Ethylenediamines	Pryilamine	Nisaval
		Tripelennamine	PBZ
II	Ethanolamines	Carbinoxamine	Clistin
		Clemastine	Tavist
		Diphenhydramine	Benadryl
III	Alkylamines	Brompheniramine	Dimetane
		Chlorpheniramine	ChlorzTrimeton
		Dexchlorpheniramine	Polaramine
		Triprolidine	Actidil
IV	Piperazines	Hydroxyzine	Atarax
		Cetirizine(*)	
V	Piperidines	Astemizole	Hismanal
		Azatadine	Optimine
		Cyproheptadine	Periactin
		Ketotifen(*)	
		Loratadine	Claritin
VI	Phenothiazines	Promethazine	Phenergan
VII	Butyrophenones	Terfenadine	Seldane
VIII	Others	Azelastine(*)	

*These are newly developed medications that have not yet become available in the United States.

Let's look at this table in more detail:

Chemical Name of Class. Antihistamines are chemicals, and all chemicals are combinations of molecules. Antihistamines have a common molecular structure to which or from which different molecules are added or subtracted to make the different antihistamine classes and agents within a class. The chemical name of each class denotes the name used by chemists, pharmacists, or doctors to describe the molecular structure common to each of the antihistaminic agents in that class. It is modifications of this common structure that make members of the same class unique. Some people think that all antihistamines are the same, but nothing could be further from the truth. Knowing the difference between types of antihistamines available will help you find the effective relief you seek.

Generic Name. Within each of seven core structures or "scaffoldings" for antihistamines, more than one variation of that structure is possible. Whenever changes are made in the core structure, the resulting antihistamine is different from any of the others in its class. This difference is recognized by giving it a name unique to itself a generic name.

Manufacturer's or Common Name. This is the trade name of the product. It is the name that appears on the package or the label of your prescription. For example, table 11-2 lists the generic name of one class CII antihistamine as being diphenhydramine. The manufacturer's name (common name, trade name) is Benadryl.

The Pros and Cons of Generic Drugs
If you ever ask a pharmacist to give you a generic instead of the manufacturer's name on your prescription, what you have actually asked the pharmacist to do is to look at the manufacturer's name on your prescription, determine what the generic name of that antihistamine actually is, and then issue you the same generic-name antihistamine in a less expensive form. Your generic will have a different manufacturer's name than your original prescription, but it will, in fact, be the exact same antihistamine. If it isn't the same generic name, you did not get exactly what your doctor wanted you to have, and you should not accept it unless your doctor has OK'd the change.

A Word About Over-The-Counter Antihistamines

If you want to purchase an over-the-counter medication, take this book with you to the drugstore. Look up the ingredients of the medicine you think you want, and assess its side-effects and cautions. This will help you make a more informed decision regarding which medication is best for you. It is always best for you to check all medications with your physician before using them.

Adverse Reactions to Antihistamines

Most of us associate antihistamines with relief of nasal symptoms. Regrettably, many of us also associate antihistamines with sleepiness, blurred vision, fatigue, nervousness, dry mouth, stomach cramps, or reduced ability to urinate.

Histamine acts on tissues only through histamine receptors. Since histamine receptors are essentially everywhere in our bodies—brains, gastrointestinal tract, urinary system, skin, lungs, and elsewhere—we can experience side effects from the use of antihistamines in a variety of ways. Even though you are taking the antihistamine for your nose symptoms, it is absorbed from your stomach and distributed to all of the tissues of your body. Not only will it act on your nose, but it may act anywhere else in your body where there are histamine receptors.

Not everyone who takes antihistamines experiences side effects, but many do. The most common side effect is drowsiness. For some, this side effect is so intolerable that they must stop taking the antihistamine. Whether or not you experience a side effect and which side effect you will experience depends upon which antihistamine preparation you take.

General Side Effects

Let's examine in more detail some of the side effects that can occur as a result of taking antihistamines:

Allergic Reactions. These include swelling of the limbs, skin, and voice box; hives; eczema (a red, dry, itchy, scaly, weeping rash); shock; and sun sensitivity.

Blood Cell Reactions. Anemia, low blood platelets, a low white blood cell count, and a reduction of all cells can occur from taking antihistamines.

Cardiovascular Reactions. These include low blood pressure upon standing; skipping, racing, irregular heart beats; fainting; increased blood pressure; EKG changes; and cardiac arrest (after injections of antihistamines).

Gastrointestinal (GI) Reactions. A variety of GI symptoms can occur from the use of antihistamines. These include abdominal cramps, nausea, and constipation. These are especially common as a result of taking class I antihistamines.

Weight gain and increased appetite may result from taking cyproheptadine (Periactin) and astemizole (Hismanal), both class V antihistamines.

Nervous System. The most common of all neurologic reactions to antihistamines is drowsiness. It is usually mild and passes after two weeks of treatment. However, due to individual variation in response to antihistamine, some find this side effect intolerable.

Other nervous system abnormalities can occur with the use of antihistamines, but they are infrequent. These include confusion, restlessness, excitation, nervousness, seizures, headache, insomnia, euphoria, and a very unusual form of muscular spasms of the neck, face, mouth, and eye muscles.

Class-Specific Side Effects

Let's look at the characteristic side effects of each class of antihistamines.

Class I: The Ethylenediamines. Sleepiness and gastrointestinal (loss of appetite, cramping) side effects are common with the use of this class of antihistamines.

Class II: The Ethanolamines. Sleepiness is a common side effect of this group. Drying of the mouth and nose, difficulty urinating, gastrointestinal cramping, and loss of appetite also occur.

Class III: The Alkylamines. These drugs are not as apt to cause sleepiness or drowsiness as most of the other classes of antihistamines. Nervousness (restlessness, irritability, excitement) is a more common side effect of this class of drugs.

Class IV: The Piperazines. Hydroxyzine by far is the most commonly used member of this class and has a marked tendency to cause sleepiness and drowsiness. Hydroxyzine has strong anti-itch properties, however.

Class V: The Piperidines. In general, these have a very low incidence of side effects because they do not tend to enter the brain (to be explained below) as readily as some of the other antihistamines. Also, there is a lower incidence of dry mouth and nose, urinary difficulty, gastrointestinal symptoms, sleepiness, and nervousness with the use of this class. Cyproheptadine and astemizole are unique to the class in their ability to cause an increased appetite.

Class VI: The Phenothiazines. This class of antihistamines is known for its ability to dry secretions and cause drowsiness or sleepiness.

Class VII: The Butyrophenones. This class is noted for its lack of sedation, due to its inability to enter the brain. Its most common side effect is headache, which occurs in a small percentage of users.

Class VIII: The Others. This is a catch-all class that has no common characteristics. All antihistamines that do not fit into any of the other classes are grouped here.

Minimizing Side Effects

Side effects of antihistamines can be minimized in these ways:

1. Take the proper dose. Do not increase the recommended dose without your physician's advice.
2. When using liquid preparations, measure doses accurately.
3. Swallow sustained/timed-release tablets or capsules whole. Do not divide or chew them.
4. If you miss a dose, do not double the next dose.
5. Most should be taken with food or fluids (milk, water, etc.) to minimize gastrointestinal side effects.

Absorption Of Antihistamines

Most antihistamines are well absorbed after being taken by mouth. However, they don't work as fast as some people think. They begin acting 15 to 30 minutes after being taken, and their maximal effects are reached in 1 to 2 hours. In general, antihistamine products not specially adapted for sustained or timed release are effective for only about 4 to 6 hours. With these products, four doses a day are required in order to maintain effective antihistamine action 24 hours a day.

This is not the case with antihistamine products that are modified to have a more sustained or timed release. These agents are effective for 8 to 24 hours, depending on the product, permitting once or twice daily dosage (Table 11-3). Claritin and Hismanal are the only not specially formulated antihistamines currently available that permit once daily dosing. However, for small children, few sustained-release products are available.

TABLE 11-3
Commonly Used Antihistamine Products: Dosing Frequency

Manufacturer's Name	Dosing Frequency
Atarax (hydroxyzine)	3 to 4 times daily
Benadryl (diphenhydramine)	3 to 4 times daily
Chlor-Trimeton (chlorpheniramine)	4 to 6 times daily
Claritin (loratadine)	once daily
Hismanal (astemizole)	once daily
PBZ (tripelennamine)	4 to 6 times daily
Seldane (terfenadine)	2 times daily
Tavist, Tavist-I (clemastine)	2 to 3 times daily

Metabolism Of Antihistamines

Most antihistamines, after being absorbed into your body, circulate to the different areas of your body where they work. How long they work in your nose varies among the antihistamine classes, and even among members of a class. Table 11-3 shows several commonly used antihistamine products and how long they might work to ease your nose symptoms.

Contraindications To The Use Of Antihistamines

The term *contraindication* refers to any situation or circumstance in which the use of a medication would be inadvisable. For most antihistamines, these cases would include the following:

- Hypersensitivity (allergy) to the medication
- Newborn and premature infants
- Nursing mothers
- Narrow-angle glaucoma
- Certain types of peptic ulcers
- Prostatic hypertrophy
- Acute asthma attacks
- Bladder neck obstruction
- Obstruction of the stomach
- Any patient taking monoamine oxidase inhibitor medications (Eutonyl, Nardil, Parnate, etc.)

- For class VII antihistamines (like Phenergan):
  Do not give to a comatose patient.
  Do not take in conjunction with barbiturates, general anesthesia, tranquilizers, alcohol, narcotics, or narcotic analgesics.
  Do not take if you have had a prior adverse reaction to a class VII antihistamine.
  Do not give to acutely ill or dehydrated children.
- For Seldane and Hismanal:
  Do not take with the antifungal agents ketoconazole (Nizoral) or itraconazole (Sporanox); with the antibiotics azithromycin (Zithromax), clarithromycin (Biaxin), erythromycin (any product), or troleandomycin (TOA). Do not take if you have liver disease or abuse alcohol. Let your physician know if you have a heart problem. Do not take more than the dose recommended by your physician.

WARNING!

Some medications are not compatible for a variety of reasons. Medications that should not be used at the same time as antihistamines are shown in table 11-4. You should *always* consult your doctor or pharmacist before taking *any* medication, and this is also true if you want to take more than one medication at a time. You should also alert your physician if you notice any unusual side effects while on any medication.

TABLE 11-4
Medications That Should Not Be Taken at the Same Time That You Are Taking Antihistamines

Alcohol, or any form of tranquilizer or sedative

Monamine oxidase inhibitor medications of any type (Eutonyl Filmtabs, Nardil, and Parnate are common products)

Phenothiazine antihistamines (Phenergan, Temaril, Tacaryl are commonly used examples) should be used with caution by patients with cardiovascular diseases, ulcers, liver diseases, or seizure disorders.

Antibiotics & Antifungals: Seldane and Hismanal contain "Block box" warnings in their product information sheets. These warnings state that rare cases of cardiovascular adverse effects have been observed by patients taking the antifungal agents ketoconazole (Nizoral) or itraconazole (Sporanox) or with the antibodics azithromycin (Zithromax), erythromycin (E-Mycin, EES, Ilosone, etc.), clarithromycin (Biaxin), or troleandomycin (TAO). Because of the close similarity between antifungal medications, they should also not be used with Diflucan (fluconazole), Flagyl (metronidazole), and intravenous Monistate (miconazole). They should not be taken in the presence of liver disease.

In addition to the above cautions, do not take antihistamines without talking with your doctor if you are pregnant or are breast feeding, have ulcers, diabetes, any urinary tract problems, a seizure disorder, or glaucoma.

THE NEW GENERATION ANTIHISTAMINES

The term *new generation antihistamines* refers to the development of four new antihistamines that, in contrast to prior antihistamines, cause little or no drowsiness. The generic names for these new products are as follows:

Astemizole   Cetirizine
Loratadine   Terfenadine

Only terfenadine (Seldane) and astemizole (Hismanal) are available in the United States at this writing. They fit into classes V and VII as shown in table 11-2.

The new generation antihistamines do not cause drowsiness because they are made in such a way that they cannot accumulate in the brain. Thus, they can't act on the histamine receptors in this area and can't make you drowsy. In addition, these antihistamines have little if any effect on the gastrointestinal tract, so abdominal cramping, nausea, and reduced appetite are uncommon.

Characteristics Of The New Generation Antihistamines

These new generation antihistamines vary considerably, as shown below, in how long each takes to clear from the body. Here's a closer look at each of these new antihistamines:

Astemizole. A member of the class V antihistamine group and metabolized by the liver, astemizole stands out as the member of the group that lasts the longest in the body: allergy skin tests can be inhibited as long as six weeks after stopping the medication. It should be stopped for four months before attempting to get pregnant. Astemizole's rate of absorption is significantly slowed if it is taken with food. In fact, it should be taken at least 2 hours after a meal or at least 1 hour before the next meal for best results. Astemizole is available in the United States and Canada under the trade name of **Hismanal**. **Warning:** Astemizole (Hismanal) should not be taken with any erythromycin product, Biaxin (clarithromycin), Zithromax (azithromycin), TAO (troleandomycin), Nizoral (ketoconazole) or Sporanox (itraconazole). Because of the close similarity between antifungal medications, it should not be used with Diflucan (fluconazole), Flagyl (metronidazole), and intravenous Monistat (miconazole). It should not be taken in the presence of liver disease. The recommended dose of 10mg daily must not be exceeded.

Cetirizine. A member of the class IV antihistamine group, cetirizine is unique among the new generation antihistamines in that it is not metabolized in the liver. In fact, it is eliminated slowly, and is unchanged in the urine. Because it is eliminated from the body through the kidney, in the presence of kidney disease (reduced kidney function), its dose should be reduced to prevent excessive accumulation in the body. Doctors usually prescribe it once daily. Unlike the other new generation antihistamines, Cetirizine can cause drowsiness. It is not available in the United States as of this writing, but it is being studied and may be available soon.

Loratadine. A member of the class V antihistamine group and metabolized by the liver, loratadine too is eliminated relatively slowly from the body Doctors usually prescribe it once daily.Of the three available new generation antihistamines loratadine is not contraindicated in patients taking erythromycin products, ketoconazole (Nizoral), itraconazole (Sporanox), clarithromycin (Biaxin), azithromycin (Zithromax), other antifungal agents, or in patients with liver disease. A study conducted in 12 healthy volunteers showed that when loratadine was taken with ketoconazole, that levels of loratadine increased. There were no significant differences in clinical adverse events between loratadine tablet groups with or without ketoconazole. However, Loratadine should be administered with caution in patients taking these medications or in the presence of liver disease. The most commonly reported side effects in clinical trials were: headache, occuring with 12% of people, drowsiness (8%), fatigue (4%), and dry mouth (3%); the same rates as in people taking placebo (sugar pill). Loratadine is available under the trade name **Claritin**.

Terfenadine. A member of the class VII antihistamine group and metabolized by the liver, terfenadine is cleared rapidly enough from the body to require twice daily administration. Terfenadine is the most widely prescribed antihistamine worldwide and has been available in the United States for several years under the trade name of Seldane. **Warning:** Terfenadine (Seldane) should not be taken with any erythromycin product, Biaxin (clarithromycin) Zithromax (azithromycin), TAO (troleandomycin), Nizoral (ketoconazole) or Sporanox (itraconazole). Because of the close similarity between antifungal medications, it should not be used with Diflucan (fluconazole), Flagyl (metronidazole), and intravenous Monistat (miconazole). It should not be taken in the presence of liver disease. The recommended dose of 60mg daily must not be exceeded.

QUESTIONS AND ANSWERS

1. Can you become "immune" to antihistamines?

No, but you can become what is called "tolerant," which means that the dose of antihistamine that once worked well for you no longer works. This reaction doesn't constitute immunity; it is only temporary. If this should happen to you, a change to another class of antihistamine should eliminate the problem. After a few weeks, you should be able to return to your former antihistamine, if you wish.

2. Are there any antihistamines that won't make it difficult for me to urinate?

The new generation antihistamines would be less likely to cause this problem, but I've seen patients who had this trouble from these as well. If you have had urinary problems with older antihistamines, a trial of one of the new generation products may be worthwhile.

3. My eyes seem to bother me more than my nose. Will antihistamines help me?

In most people with nasal allergy, nose irritations dominate their symptoms. However, in some people, the nasal symptoms are minor compared to the eye symptoms. Fortunately for these people, antihistamines in general work very well in the relief of red, watery, and itchy eyes.

4. I've heard that if you have asthma, you shouldn't take antihistamines. Is this true?

Most people with asthma can take antihistamines, but there are two reasons why so many packages instruct asthma sufferers not to use antihistamines: (1) to discourage patients from trying to use antihistamines to treat their own asthma (they don't work well for asthma), and (2) because, *theoretically*, these drugs can dry mucus, thus making it difficult for patients with asthma to expel mucus from their airways. Thus far, there is no evidence that these agents actually do cause drying of the airway sufficiently to cause any difficulty in the handling of airway mucus by patients with asthma, although it is possible that there is a small subset of patients with asthma who do experience difficulty in coughing up mucus when using antihistamines.

CHAPTER 12

THE NASAL DECONGESTANTS

ANTIHISTAMINES ARE WONDERFUL drugs for sneezing, itching, runny noses, drainage, and very mild nasal congestion. However, when nasal stuffiness or congestion is a major part of your symptoms, you should turn to or include a decongestant for relief.

THE BASICS OF DECONGESTANTS

How Decongestants Work

Most of the nasal congestion or stuffiness you experience results from a combination of events that cause the lining of the nose to become swollen: (1) dilation of the blood vessels in the lining of your nose thickens the lining membrane, and (2) leakage of blood plasma from blood vessels into the tissue around the vessels swells the lining where the leaking has occurred. Both of these events are the result of histamine acting on histamine receptors in the cells lining the blood vessel walls and on the tiny muscles that encircle the vessels. These two events cause the lining of the nose to swell, which reduces the size of the passageway for air, causing a stuffy or stopped-up nose.

Like antihistamines, decongestants act through receptors. The interaction of decongestant and receptor causes blood vessels to constrict, halting the oozing of plasma from the blood vessels into the tissue. After the nasal membrane swelling ceases, the membranes shrink, allowing more room in the nose for air to pass. Thus, your nose becomes "open" once again. Decongestants were developed because, although antihistamines are very good at reducing runny nose, sneezing, postnasal drainage, and itching of the nose, throat, and roof of the mouth, they aren't good at decongesting noses. Since many people who suffer from a nose problem have congestion as well as runny noses, sneezing, etc., many commonly used prescription and nonprescription nasal medications contain both an antihistamine and a decongestant.

Types Of Decongestants

There are two general types of decongestants: topical decongestants and systemic decongestants.

Topical Decongestants. These are sprayed or dropped into the nose. They work within a few minutes because they are placed directly into the nose.

Systemic Decongestants. These are tablets, liquids, or capsules taken by mouth. They do not work as quickly because they must first be absorbed into the blood, circulated to the tissues, and taken up by the tissues where they can then begin to work. Since they circulate in the blood before arriving at the nose, tissues other than the nose can take in decongestants. It's because of their ability to act in tissues other than the nose that you notice more side effects with systemic decongestants than with topical decongestant sprays or drops. Their advantage over topical decongestants is that they do not cause rebound or chemical rhinitis (chapter 9).

In addition, there are different types of topical and different types of systemic decongestants. Tables 12-1 and 12-3 show the more common forms of both types, giving their chemical names, common names, and length of time they tend to work in the nose. These tables should make clear that if one decongestant preparation doesn't work, others are available that may do the trick.

The Topical Decongestants: Sprays and Drops

While nose drops and sprays offer the advantages of working quickly and effectively, they have the potential for causing rebound nasal congestion if used for longer than 3 to 5 days.

Indications for topical nasal decongestants. The best use of these decongestants is for temporary relief of nasal stuffiness or congestion due to most forms of allergic and nonallergic rhinitis. In addition, they can be useful in the treatment of infected sinuses and ears, as well as Eustachian tube blockage (the tube that connects the nose cavity to the middle ear) malfunction, which will be discussed in more detail when we talk about fluid in the ears and infected ears, a complication of having rhinitis.

How often to use nasal sprays or drops. Table 12-1 can help here. Notice that there is a column marked "Duration of Action." That term indicates approximately how long the agent(s) work in the nose. For example, the table shows that NeoSynephrine drops and sprays work for about 1 to 4 hours. Therefore, they will probably have to be used several times a day to keep your nose open. In contrast, Afrin, Dristan Long Lasting, or Duration work for 5 to 12 hours and are recommended to be used only twice daily. There is no advantage to the use of short-acting nasal decongestants sprays or drops.

A Word of Advice: Whenever you use topical nasal decongestants, always check the package for instructions regarding how many sprays or drops should be used with each treatment, how many times a day treatments should be taken, and for how many days the product can be used.

TABLE 12-1
The Topical Decongestants:
Commonly Used Nasal Sprays and Nasal Drops

Generic Name	Common Name	Duration of Action
Ephedrine	Vatronol	1 to 4 hours
Phenylephrine	Alconefrin 12	
	Duration	
	Neo-Synephrine	1 to 4 hours
	Nostril	
	Rhinall	
	Sinex	
Naphazoline	Privine	2 to 6 hours
Oxymetazoline	Afrin	
	Afrin Childrens	
	Allerest	12 Hour
	Coricidin	5 to 12 hours
	Dristan Long Lasting	
	Duration	
	4-Way Long Acting	
	Sinex Long Acting	
Xylometazoline	Otrivin Drops	6 to 12 hours
	Otrivin Pediatric	

Side Effects of Nasal Sprays and Drops. The possible side effects caused by nasal sprays or drops usually are limited to the nose. The most troublesome is rebound swelling of the nasal lining or chemical rhinitis, as discussed earlier. Other side effects include burning and stinging inside the nose and the sensation of a dry nose. However, generalized side effects can occur from nasal sprays and drops if the medication is absorbed into your bloodstream. These are the same kinds of side effects that you could experience after taking a decongestant liquid, tablet, or capsule, as discussed below.

Contraindications to Use of Topical Decongestant Sprays or Drops
• If you are allergic (itch, rash, wheeze, flush, etc.) to the spray or drop to be used
• If you have experienced uncomfortable side effects from

the medication with prior use
*   If you have health problems that could be aggravated by the use of decongestants (see cautions section, below)
*   On your infant or a young child (except under the direction of your child's physician)
*   If you have been using a nasal spray or drops, but they are no longer working (you're suffering from rebound; call your doctor for instructions)

Nasal decongestant sprays and drops are generally safe and effective medications, but a few tips regarding their use are worth mentioning (Table 12-2):

TABLE 12-2
Tips for the Safe Use of
Nasal Decongestant Sprays and Drops

Use the lowest dose that is effective as directed on the package.

Use for no more than 3 to 5 days without discussing with your doctor.

If medication hasn't worked well in two to three days, or if your symptoms are worsening, call your doctor for additional advice.

Do not use in young children except under the supervision of a physician.

The Right Way to Take Topical Nasal Decongestants. Most people take these medications incorrectly. Here is the correct procedure:
*   **Nasal Drops.** Lie down on your left or right side, with your head lower than the rest of your body. Put the drops into the side of the nose on which you are lying. For example, if you are lying on your left side, put the drops in your left nostril. Stay in this position 2 to 3 minutes. Then roll over, and repeat the process on the other side of your nose.
*   **Nasal Sprays.** Spray one side of your nose while sitting or standing. Then, lie down on that side with your head lower

than the rest of your body. Stay in this position 2 to 3 minutes. Then get up, spray the other side of your nose, and repeat the lying-down process on the other side.

It is much more convenient for working people to select one of the longer-acting preparations so that these procedures can be done before and after going to work.

The Systemic Decongestants: The Pills and Capsules

Decongestants taken by mouth are available in a variety of forms: liquids, tablets, and timed-release capsules and tablets. This diversity of forms permits accurate dosage for all ages and permits flexibility in the frequency of doses (liquids and tablets usually are taken 4 times a day; timed-release capsules and tablets usually are taken 2 times a day).

Table 12-3 lists some of the more commonly used oral decongestant medications. They are variations of only two generic products: pseudoephedrine and phenylpropanolamine.

TABLE 12-3
The Systemic Decongestants:
Commonly Used Liquids, Pills, and Capsules

Generic Name	Common Name	Duration Of Action
Pseudoephedrine liquid	Sudafed	1-4 hours
Pseudoephedrine tablets 30mg	Sudafed	
Pseudoephedrine tablets 60mg	Sudafed	
Pseudoephedrine caps/tabs timed release 120mg	Sudafed 12 Hour	6-8 hours
Phenylpropanolamine 25mg	Propagest	1-4 hours
Phenylpropanolamine 50mg	Maigret-50	
Phenylpropanolamine 75mg timed release	Rhindecon	6-8 hours

Pseudoephedrine, in one form or another, is by far the most commonly used systemic decongestant preparation. **Phenyl-**

propanolamine is used less often as a decongestant. In fact, it is more commonly used as an over-the-counter "diet pill" because of its side effect: appetite reduction.

When to Use a Systemic Decongestant. Systemic decongestants are the "drugs of choice" for decongesting most noses. Like topical decongestants, they are also used in the treatment of infected ears and sinuses, and in ear-tube malfunction.

Some people take oral decongestants before traveling in airplanes in order to lessen ear problems that can occur with changes in altitude. Whereas nasal decongestant drops and sprays should never be used for longer than a few days, the systemic decongestants can be used for longer periods of time. It is not uncommon for someone with chronic rhinitis to take these medications on a daily basis for weeks or months. They rarely cause rebound nasal congestion.

Side Effects Caused by Systemic Decongestants. Side effects are more common and potentially more serious with the systemic decongestants than with topical decongestants since they are taken by mouth, and since the dosage required for effectiveness is much higher than that required if the medication is sprayed or dropped directly onto the lining of the nose. Once medications enter the blood, they may affect areas other than the nose, such as the heart, blood pressure, urinary tract, stomach, eyes, and brain.

CAUTIONS WHEN USING ANY KIND
OF DECONGESTANT

General Cautions

If you are allergic to a decongestant or if you just cannot tolerate its side effects, don't take it!

Excessive and repeated use of nasal sprays or drops should be avoided as they cause rebound nasal congestion, known as chemical rhinitis.

Finally, if you're not sleeping well, it could be the decongestant you're taking. They can cause insomnia.

Age Cautions

Infants and Young Children. Nasal decongestant drops and/or sprays should not be used in infants or small children, except under the supervision of a physician.

Adults over Sixty Years. If you are over sixty, you are more likely to experience a side effect from a decongestant. In addition, that side effect is likely to be more severe than if you were younger

Sex Cautions

Pregnancy Cautions. The effects on the developing fetus are always of concern. Use these agents in pregnancy only after seeking advice from a health professional.

Lactation Cautions. Phenylpropanolamine is not recommended for use by nursing mothers.

Disease Cautions

Do not take decongestants if you have **high blood pressure or heart problems** without talking with your doctor.

Patients with **enlarged prostates** should use decongestants with caution.

Patients with **diabetes** should use decongestants with caution, as they can cause an elevation of blood sugar.

If you have **hyperthyroidism**, decongestants can increase your discomfort.

Cautions Relating To Other Medications When Taken With Decongestants

Heart/Blood Pressure Medications. Patients using **Beta blockers** could experience abnormal heart rhythms and increased blood pressure. These types of medications include Corgard, Corzide, Inderal, Lopressor, Normodyne, Tinormin.

Guanethidine may lose its effect if taken with deconges-tants. Medications containing guanethidine include Esimil and Ismelin.

Parkinsons Disease Medications. Use with *Methyldopa* may cause abnormally high blood pressure to develop. Medica-tions containing methyldopa include Aldoclor, Aldomet, Aldoril, and Methyidopa.

Phenothiazines. Use with these could cause abnormally low blood pressure to develop. Common phenothiazine medications include Compazine, Mellaril, Thorazine, Triavil.

Theophylline. Use with these may cause GI distress and nervousness. Common theophylline products include Theo-Dur, Slo-Phyllin, and Slo-bid.

Tricyclic antidepressants. Use with these could increase blood pressure. These medications include Elavil, Endep, Pamelor, Sinequan, Tofranil.

Cautions Concerning Specific Decongestant Medications

Naphazoline should not be used if you have glaucoma.

Phenylpropanolamine is best not used by nursing mothers or children under 12 years. It should also be avoided if you have high blood pressure. If a decongestant is needed, a pseudoephedrine product should be used.

QUESTIONS AND ANSWERS

1. Every time I fly, my ears clog and hurt for several days. Is there anything I can do to help this?

There are several remedies you can try. First, use a topical, long-acting nasal decongestant spray about 30 minutes before you get on the airplane. Frequently, just doing this will resolve the problem. Instead of or in addition to using the nasal spray, you also could take a long-acting pseudoephedrine preparation about 90 minutes before your flight.

2. I understand why people with heart and blood pressure problems should be careful when using decongestants, but why the warning for people with diabetes?

One of the non-nasal actions of decongestants is to release sugar or glucose from storage in the liver and muscles. When this happens, the blood sugar level rises. A rise in blood sugar can worsen diabetes.

3. I have tried three different decongestants and none of them has worked. Am I "immune" to decongestants?

We don't become "immune" to decongestants. If nasal congestion is one of your main symptoms and decongestants in proper doses don't help, there are many other options. What you need most at this point is a diagnosis by a doctor of the cause of your symptoms. Once that is done, other treatment options can be made available.

4. Every time I take pseudoephedrine 60 milligram tablets, I develop difficulty urinating. Which decongestants won't do this?

Any decongestant taken by mouth can do this. If you are using pseudoephedrine, then you might try a phenylpropanotamine preparation, and visa versa, to see if both types affect you. If you need a decongestant infrequently, and only for a few days at a time, use a topical decongestant, as they do not cause this side effect.

5. Which form of decongestant should I use: nose sprays, nose drops, liquids, pills, or capsules?

Nasal sprays or drops should be used when your symptoms require short-term treatment of no more than a few days. These medications can last from just over 1 hour to 12 hours, depending on the product you choose. Never use these longer than a few days.

Liquids are mainly used in children, although occasionally an adult will prefer to take liquids rather than pills. Liquids generally taste good and give the doctor enough flexibility to safely and effectively dose almost any size child. As an added bonus, liquids permit dosing of children and adults who cannot or will not swallow tablets or capsules. A disadvantage of liquid decongestants is that they do not act long in the body, and usually require doses 4 times a day.

Tablets come in two forms: rapid release and sustained or timed release. The rapid-release tablets get into your system and act quickly and generally lose potency within 4 hours. The sustained-release tablets release their medication slowly, thereby maintaining effectiveness for several hours (6 to 8 hours).

CHAPTER 13

TAKING PRESCRIPTION
ANTIHISTAMINE-DECONGESTANT
MEDICATIONS SAFELY

IF YOU HAVE NASAL STUFFINESS or congestion in addition to other nasal symptoms (runny nose, postnasal drainage, sneezing, etc.), then you may need a medication that contains *both* an antihistamine and a decongestant. Such medications are called combination products. Such *combination products* are available both by prescription as well as over-the-counter (OTC). This chapter is about prescription combination medications. Nonprescription combination products will be discussed in chapter 14.

Prescription Antihistamine-Decongestant Combinations

Below are listings of the more commonly prescribed antihistamine-decongestant combination products (tables 13-1 through 13-3). Listed first are the combination products that do not last very long in the body and that generally require dosing more than twice each day to control symptoms. These are known as the *rapid-release combination products.* These commonly exist as liquids and tablets.

The Rapid-Release Combinations

Liquids. Children benefit from antihistamine-decongestant medications just as do adults. However, many cannot take tablets or capsules. The availability of liquid preparations makes it possible for children to receive accurate and effective doses of these medications.

TABLE 13-1
Commonly Used Prescription Rapid-Release
Combination Liquid Products*

(Note: all doses are provided in ml/teaspoon)

Brand Name	Active Agent
Deconamine Syrup	2mg chlorpheniramine (A)
	30mg pseudoephedrine (D)
ChemTuss Elixir	4mg chlorpheniramine (A)
	10mg phenylephrine (D)
Histalet Syrup	3mg chlorpheniramine (A)
	45mg pseudoephedrine (D)
Naldecon Syrup	7.5mg phenyltoloxamine (A)
	5mg phenylephrine (D)
Naldecon Pediatric Syrup	0.5mg chlorpheniramine (A)
	2mg phenyltoloxamine (A)
	5mg phenylpropanolamine (D)
	1.25mg phenylephrine (D)
Phenergan VC Syrup	6.25mg promethazine (A)
	5mg phenylephrine (D)
Poly-Histine-D Elixir	4mg pyrilamine (A)
	4mg phenyltoloxamine (A)
	4mg pheniramine (A)
	12.5mg phenylpropanolamine (D)
Rondec Syrup	2mg carbinoxamine (A)
	25mg ˙ pseudoephedrine (D)

(A) Antihistamine, (D) Decongestant

Tablets. For many adults and older children, the rapid-release antihistamine-decongestant formulations offer the best combination of dose and frequency of administration.

TABLE 13-2
Commonly Used Prescription
Rapid-Release Combination Tablets*
(Note: all doses are provided in mg/tablets)

Brand Name	Active Agents
Actihist Tablets	2.5mg triprolidine (A)
	60mg pseudoephedrine (D)
Bromfed Tablets	4mg brompheniramine (A)
	60mg pseudoephedrine (D)
Comhist Tablets	2mg chlorpheniramine (A)
	25mg phenyltoloxamine (A)
	10mg phenylephrine (D)
Deconarnine Tablets	4mg chlorpheniramine (A)
	60mg pseudoephedrine (D)
Hista-Vadrin Tablets	6mg chlorpheniramine (A)
	40mg phenylpropanolamine (D)
	5mg phenylephrine (D)
Histalet Forte Tablets	6mg chlorpheniramine (A)
	50mg phenylpropanolamine (D)
	5mg phenylephrine (D)
Phenergan-D Tablets	6.25mg promethazine (A)
	60mg pseudoephedrine (D)
Rondec Tablets	4mg carbinoxamine (A)
	60mg pseudoephedrine (D)
Rynatan Tablets	8mg chlorpheniramine (A)
	25mg pyrilamine (A)
	25mg phenylephrine (D)

(A) Antihistamine, (D) Decongestant

As you can see, brompheniramine and chlorpheniramine are the two antihistamines used most commonly in the rapid release combination products. Therefore, if you change products because the one you are using is not working, be sure that the product you switch to has a different antihistamine content, otherwise the only change you will make will be name, color, form, and shape, but not content.

The Sustained-Release Combination Products

Listed next (table 13-3) will be those products that last longer in the body and usually require only twice a day dosing: *sustained release combination products.* These generally exist as tablets and capsules, with the exception of Rynatan Pediatric Suspension. It is a sustained-release liquid.

TABLE 13-3
Commonly Used Prescription
Sustained-Release Combination Products*
(Note: all doses are in mg/tablet or capsule)

Brand Name	Active Agents
Atrohist Sprinkle Caps	2mg brompheniramine (A)
	25mg phenyltoloxaniine (A)
	10mg phenylephrine (D)
Brexin	8mg chlorpheniramine (A)
	120mg pseudoephedrine (D)
Bromfed Capsules	12mg brompheniramine (A)
	120mg pseudoephedrine (D)
Bromfed-PD Capsules	6mg brompheniramine (A)
	60mg pseudoephedrine (D)
ChemTuss SR Tablets	8mg chlorpheniramine (A)
	25mg phenylephrine (D)
	50mg phenylpropanolamine (D)
Comhist LA Capsules	4mg chlorpheniramine (A)
	50mg phenyltoloxamine (A)
	20mg phenylephrine (D)
Cophene No. 2 Capsules	12mg chlorpheniraniine (A)
	120mg pseudoephedrine (D)
Dallergy-JR Capsules	6mg brompheniramine (A)
	60mg pseudoephedrine (D)
Deconamine SR Capsules	8mg chlorpheniramine (A)
	120mg pseudoephedrine (D)
Fedahist Timecaps	8mg chlorpheniramine (A)
	120mg pseudoephedrine (D)

Fedahist Gyrocaps	8mg chlorpheniramine (A)
	65mg pseudoephedrine (D)
Histaspan-Plus Capsules	8mg chlorpheniramine (A)
	20mg phenylephrine (D)
Isoclor Timesules	8mg chlorpheniramine (A)
	120mg pseudoephedrine (D)
Kronofed-A Kronocaps	8mg chlorpheniramine (A)
	120mg pseudoephedrine (D)
Kronofed-A-Jr. Kronocaps	4mg chlorpheniramine (A)
	60mg pseudoephedrine (D)
Naldecon Tablets	5mg chlorpheniraniine (A)
	15mg phenyltoloxamine (A)
	40mg phenylpropanolamine (D)
	10mg phenylephrine (D)
Novafed-A Capsules	8mg chlorpheniramine (A)
	120mg pseudoephedrine (D)
Ornade Spansuies	12mg chlorpheniraniine (A)
	75mg pseudoephedrine (D)
Rondec-TR Tablets	8mg carbinoxamine (A)
	120mg pseudoephedrine (D)
Ru-Tuss II Capsules	12mg chlorpheniramine (A)
	75mg phenylpropanolamine (D)
Rynatan	8mg chlorpheniramine (A)
	25mg pyrilamine (A)
	25mg phenylephrine (D)
Rynatan Pediatric Suspension	2mg chlorpheniramine (A)
	12.5mg pyritamine (A)
	5mg pseudoephedrine (D)
Seldane-D	60mg terfenadine (A)
	120mg pseudoephedrine (D)
Tavist-D Tablets	1.34mg clemastine (A)
	120mg pseudoephedrine (D)
Triaminic TR Tablets	25mg pyrilamine (A)
	25mg pheniramine (A)
	50mg phenylpropanolamine (D)
Trinaline Repetabs	lmg azatadine (A)
	120mg pseudoephedrine (D)

(A) Antihistamine, (D) Decongestant

Besides listing the antihistamine and decongestant composition of commonly used products for rhinitis, this table will permit you to readily identify products that are exactly the same.

For example: Brexin, Deconamine SR Capsules, and Fedahist Timecaps, Isoclor Timesules, Kronofed-A Kronocaps, and Novafed-A Capsules each contain 8 milligrams chlorpheniramine and 120 milligrams pseudoephedrine. While their brand name, color, and form (liquid, tablet, capsule) may vary, they are the same product, should produce the same effect, cause the same types of side effects, and can be used interchangeably.

This information can make you a more informed consumer as well as save you money. Check prices before you buy. For example, when selecting from two or more products that are exactly the same ask the pharmacist which is the least expensive.

In addition, if a specific brand-name product has not worked for you, be sure that the next brand name you get is truly different in its chemical composition. For example, if Ru-Tuss II Capsules are not working or make you sleepy, you would not want to substitute Ornade Spansules, as they differ in name only.

A rapid-release medication generally provides a lower dose/tablet of both antihistamine and decongestant than would a sustained-release product. This variation can be advantageous to those bothered by side effects of either drug. The prime disadvantage of this is that, in general, the rapid-release products must be taken more than twice daily to provide consistent relief of symptoms.

Seldane-D Extended-Release Tablets is the only nonsedating antihistamine (terfenadine)-decongestant (pseudoephedrine) combination available in the United States. These tablets combine terfenadine (60 milligrams) and pseudoephedrine (120 milligrams) in an extended-release format designed to be used on a twice daily dosing schedule. The terfenadine component is contained in the outer coating of the tablet and is released immediately upon ingestion, which is fine, because its effect will last up to 12 hours. The pseudoephedrine is released in two stages. Ten milligrams is present in the outer coating and is released for immediate action along with the terfenadine. The other 110 milligrams of pseudophedrine is contained in the inner portion of the tablet and is made available slowly over several hours. The recommended dose for children over twelve years and adults is one tablet each morning and evening. The same cautions one observes in the use of either component alone should be observed when using the combination. Seldane-D carries with it the same warnings as Seldane: it should not be taken with any erythromycin product, Biaxin (clarithromycin), Zithromax (azithromycin), TAO (troleandomycin), Nizoral (ketoconazole), or Sporanox (itraconazole). Because of the close similarity between antifungal medications, it should not be used with Diflucan (fluconazole), Flagyl (metronidazole), and intravenous Monistat (miconazole). It should not be taken in the presence of liver disease. It should be taken only in the dose recommended by your physician.

QUESTIONS AND ANSWERS

1. My brother took Novafed-A Capsules and got relief for a while, but then they seemed to stop working. He changed to Fedahist Timecaps, then to Deconamine SR Capsules and finally to Kronofed-A Kronocaps, but none of them helped. Did he develop an immunity to antihistamines?

You can't become immune to antihistamines. However, if you use the same antihistamine for a prolonged period of time you may notice that it seems to be less effective. This is not an immunity because it does not involve any antibodies or other immune-system reactions. It is usually easily remedied either by increasing the dose of antihistamine (provided you are not already taking the maximum dose) or by changing to a different antihistamine. All your brother actually did was change product names (brand names) but not antihistamines. Although these medications had different brand names and colors, they each contained the same type of antihistamine. If he changes the type of antihistamine he uses, he might find relief again.

2. Why do Cophene No. 2 Capsules make me sleepy and RuTuss II Tablets make me nervous? My doctor said they were the "same thing."

They are the same only in that both contain the same dose of antihistamine—12 milligrams of chlorpheniramine—plus a decongestant. However, they are very different regarding the decongestants they contain: Cophene No. 2 contains 120 milligrams pseudoephedrine and Ru-Tuss 11 contains 75 milligrams phenylpropanolamine. It is possible for you to get very nervous from one decongestant (phenylpropanolamine) and not from the other (pseudoephedrine). In your case, the absence of side effects from the pseudoephedrine in Cophene No. 2 allows the sedation effect of the antihistamine (chlorpheniramine) to dominate the side effects you notice.

3. Fedahist Gyrocaps relieved my runny nose and sneezing, but my nose was still congested. My doctor changed me to Kronofed-A Kronocaps, and this solved my problem. What happened?

Your doctor advised you to take a stronger decongestant medication, almost double. Fedahist Gyrocaps and Kronofed-A Kronocaps both contain the same antihistamines milligrams chlorpheniramine. There was no reason to change this part of your medication as the types of symptoms antihistamines help— runny nose, sneezing, etc.—were being controlled. However, you were not getting sufficient decongestion from 65 milligrams pseudoephedrine. He prescribed another product containing the same dose of antihistamine, but a stronger dose of decongestant.

4. I am an electrical lineman, which is a hazardous occupation. I have bad hay fever and must take an antihistamine. I need a non-sedating antihistamine because it is dangerous for me to be sleepy, but the non-sedating antihistamine I take doesn't help my stopped-up nose. Can I take a decongestant medication with my non-sedating antihistamine?

Taking a decongestant with your antihistamine is a sensible choice. The stand-alone decongestants commonly available contain either pseudoephedrine or phenylpropanolamine. I generally prescribe pseudoephedrine in either 60-milligram or 120milligram sustained-release tablet forms that are scored so they can be broken in half. This permits you to take either 30 milligrams, 60 milligrams, or 120 milligrams of pseudoephedrine twice daily-whichever dose best helps your symptoms. Ask your doctor.

CHAPTER 14

TAKING OVER-THE-COUNTER NASAL MEDICATIONS SAFELY

IF YOU HAVE EVER GONE to the drugstore seeking relief for a troubled nose, no doubt you were faced with a wall of shelves full of different over-the-counter (OTC) products of varying sizes, shapes, colors, and claims and with words such as "sinus, cold, allergy, hay fever," and "no-drowsiness formula."

In the cold and nose section of any large drugstore there are likely to be over 150 different products. In fact, however, many of these products are exactly the same medication: they are simply placed in different packages, given different names, made in different forms, and colored differently. One effect of this is to give the impression to the uninformed consumer of difference where none exists. Such displays place you at a disadvantage when trying to select an OTC nose agent, because it is neither good care nor safe for the consumer to be invited to make selections in the midst of such marketing confusion.

Your Doctor And Your Pharmacist Are Your Fiends

Before we go any further, let me say this: always remember that both your doctor and your pharmacist are there to help you. If there is any question about a medication, be it prescription or OTC, ask either of them for explanations.

MEDICATIONS AND YOUR NOSE

Some 400,000 OTC products are sold to millions of Americans each year, for billions of dollars. These medications are purchased by people who frequently know little more about them than the symptoms they hope they will help.

Why Use OTC Nose Medications?

Use OTC medications because many are effective, especially on symptoms many feel are not serious enough to require a call or a visit to their doctor. All are easy to obtain and are relatively inexpensive.

You Can Learn A Lot From The Package or Box

Every OTC medication must have the following very important and helpful information printed on its package or box:
1. The name of the medication.
2. The name and address of the manufacturer, packer, or distributor.
3. How many tablets, capsules, or how much fluid is contained in the package.
4. The established pharmaceutical name of all the product's active ingredients.
5. The name of any habit-forming ingredients in the product.
6. Cautions and warnings that are necessary to protect you from harm when using the product. These tell you how to use a medication safely, when not to use the medication, when to stop taking the medication, and when you should see a physician.
7. Adequate directions for the safe and effective dosage of the medication.

When Not To Use OTC Medications

If you don't *need* it, don't take it. Very mild symptoms do not need medications. In addition, do not use OTC nasal medications if you have the following conditions:

- High blood pressure
- Angina
- Skipped beats of your heart or other heart rhythm problems
- An overactive thyroid gland
- Pain in your head or face
- Pregnant, planning to be pregnant, or are nursing
- Blowing blood or pus from your nose
- Symptoms that have been present for longer than two weeks
- Symptoms that go away but recur over and over
- Symptoms that are getting worse rather than better while taking medication
- Symptoms that include loss of hearing or pain in your ear

How To Safely And Effectively Use OTC Medications

- Be reasonably sure that your symptoms are not a reflection of something more serious.
- Select a product that will help your symptoms.
- Use products composed of only a single agent, either decongestant or antihistamine, when possible.
- Products containing two or more antihistamines are no more effective than products with a single antihistamine.
- Products containing more than one decongestant are no more effective than products with a single decongestant.
- Combination products with more than one antihistamine or decongestant are no more effective than those with a single antihistamine and a single decongestant.
- There is no advantage in adding a pain-relieving medication to either an antihistamine, a decongestant or a combination product. If you have pain with your nasal

symptoms, and do not otherwise have headaches, call your doctor.

- Do not take more medication than is suggested by the manufacturer.
- Do not take more frequently than recommended by the manufacturer.
- Take the medication you select only as long as you need it. If you need it longer than a week, however, discuss your symptoms with your doctor.
- If you are using liquids, shake them well before using and measure your doses with a standard measuring device, one that accurately measures the dose in either teaspoons or milliliters. These can be obtained from your pharmacist.

Myths About OTC Medications

You may have heard one of the following myths, but none of them is true:

MYTH: OTC medications are not as strong as prescription medications.

FACT: Many OTC medications are just as strong as prescription drugs.

MYTH: OTC medications are less expensive than prescription medications.

FACT: Check the prices.

MYTH: If one tablet, capsule, or teaspoonful works, two should work even better.

FACT: Never exceed the recommended dose!

MYTH: Rapid-release decongestant tablets taken 4 times daily affect blood pressure less than the sustained-release tablets or capsules taken twice daily

FACT: Actually, the sustained-release medications tend to affect blood pressure less.

MYTH: Because these medications are over-the-counter, they are free from danger.

FACT: They are safe only when used exactly as directed and

cautioned. These medications can aggravate blood pressure, diabetes, thyroid disease, and more. Any medication can be harmful.

MYTH: Liquid OTC medications are not strong medications.

FACT: Wrong again. Some are stronger than others, but too many teaspoons of a weak medication turns it into a strong medication.

Selecting The OTC Product That Is Best For You

Should you use a decongestant, an antihistamine, or both? And when to use which?

The first step in answering these questions is to determine which nasal symptom(s) you want to relieve. Your symptom(s) will determine whether or not you select an antihistamine product, a decongestant product, or a combination product (one composed of both types of medications). The following guide may be helpful:

Nasal Symptoms	Type of Product Needed
Congestion or stuffiness	Decongestant
Runny nose	Antihistamine
Sneezing	Antihistamine
Postnasal drip	Antihistamine
Itching of the nose	Antihistamine
Congestion or stuffiness and one or more of the other symptoms above	Antihistamine + Decongestant

NOTE: if you need a combination product, choose one that contains only *one* antihistamine and *one* decongestant.

The Most Common OTCs For Rhinitis

What follows are listings of the more common decongestant, antihistamine, and combination products available OTC. **Please note: Each product is listed according to the following:**
  • Product Name

• Active Agent(s): these can be either
Antihistamine(s), or
Decongestant(s)

If a product contains more than one active agent, like an antihistamine *and* a decongestant, both are listed.

If you need only a decongestant. Try a nasal spray or drops first. Discussed in some detail in chapter 12, the more commonly used OTC sprays are listed in table 14-1. They work quickly, with effective relief, for several hours. They do not cause significant generalized effects, and can usually be used for 3 to 5 days without the development of rebound. I most often recommend one of the long-acting decongestant sprays. This limits your choices to one of two chemical agents, each of which can last from 5 to 12 hours:

Oxymetazoline
Xylometazoline

In using long-acting nasal sprays or drops, *observe these cautions:*

• Do not use longer than 3 to 5 days without talking to your doctor
• Do not use in infants, except under the direction of your physician

The commonly used long-acting nasal decongestant sprays and drops you will likely encounter on the shelf at the drugstore are listed below in table 14-1.

TABLE 14-1
Long-Acting CVRC Decongestant Nasal Sprays*

Product Name	Active Agent
Afrin Regular Spray	0.05% oxymetazoline
Afrin Menthol Spray	0.05% oxymetazoline

TABLE 14-1 (continued)
Long-Acting OTC Decongestant Nasal Sprays*

Product Name	Active Agent
Allerest 12 Hour Spray	0.05% oxymetazoline
Coricidin Nasal Mist	0.05% oxymetazoline
Dristan Long Lasting Spray	0.05% oxymetazoline
Duration Spray	0.05% oxymetazoline
4-Way Long Acting Nasal Spray	0.05% oxymetazoline
Neo-Synephrine 12 Hour	0.05% oxymetazoline
Neo-Synephrine 12 Hour With Menthol	0.05% oxymetazoline
Nostrilla Long Acting Nasal Spray	0.05% oxymetazoline
NTZ Long Acting Nasal Spray	0.05% oxymetazoline
Otrivin Spray	0.05% oxymetazoline
Sinarest 12-Hour Spray	0.05% oxymetazoline
Sinex Long Acting	0.05% oxymetazoline

Note: There is no significant difference between these products.

A word of caution: Duration Spray also comes in a form that does not contain either oxymetazoline or xylometazoline but a shorter-acting agent. The same is true for several variations of Neo-Synephrine spray.

If you need a decongestant longer than 3 to 5 days. You will need to take one by mouth. Again, many physicians recommend a sustained-release decongestant rather than a rapid release product. Select one of the sustained-release products. Sustained-release products allow you the most convenient dosage schedule (twice a day) rather than a schedule that requires that medication be taken every 4 to 6 hours. Most twice a day medications are meant to be taken about 12 hours apart, for example at 8 AM and 8 PM. Young children, however, need liquids or tablets which require the more frequent dosing schedules.

As you will see below, most of the oral decongestants, whether rapid release or sustained release, are variations of two chemical agents:

Pseudoephedrine

Phenylpropanolamine

Commonly used sustained-release decongestant tablets or capsules available OTC in your drugstore are listed below in table 14-2.

TABLE 14-2
Sustained-Release OTC Decongestant Tablets/Capsules

Product Name	Active Agent
Afrin Tablets	120mg pseudoephedrine
Phenylpropanolamine	75mg phenylpropanolamine
Sudafed 12 Hour	120mg pseudoephedrine

If you need an antihistamine. The major concern about the use of antihistamines is that they can make you drowsy. Unfortunately, none of the three antihistamines available in the United States that do not cause drowsiness—Claritin (loratidine), Hismanal (astemizole), Seldane (terfenadine)—are available OTC.

Fortunately, not all antihistamines cause the same degree of drowsiness. For example (see table 11-2), the class II antihistamines (ethanolamines), of which diphenhydramine (Benadryl) is the most commonly used, frequently cause drowsiness. Class III antihistamines (alkylamines), on the other hand, cause drowsiness infrequently, as does a class I antihistamine (ethylenediamines) called pyrilamine (Nisalal).

The antihistamines available for OTC use least likely to cause drowsiness include brompheniramine, chlorpheniramine, clemastine, dexbrompheniramine, triprolidine, and pyrilamine. However, dexbrompheniramine and triprolidine are available only in products that also contain a decongestant (see table 14-4). Pyrilamine is available only in prescription products. Therefore, your OTC selection of a sustained-release (minimally sedating) antihistamine is limited to a product composed of one of only three chemical agents:

Brompheniramine
Chlorpheniramine
Clemastine

Commonly used OTC antihistamine sustained-release products containing brompheniramine or chlorpheniramine are listed below in table 14-3.

TABLE 14-3
Sustained-Release OTC Decongestant Tablets/Capsules

Product Name	Active Agent
Chlor-Trimeton Repetabs	8mg Chlorpheniramine
Chlor-Trimeton Repetabs	12mg Chlorpheniramine
Dimetane Extendtabs	8mg Brompheniramine
Dimetane Extendtabs	12mg Brompheniramine
Teldrin	12mg Chlorphenirarnine
Tavist-1	1.34mg Clemastine (*)

(*) Technically, this is not a sustained-release product, but it is long-acting and is commonly used in a twice daily dosing schedule.

If you need both an antihistamine and a decongestant. Your selection can be expanded to one that contains one of two decongestants:

Pseudoephedrine
Phenylpropanolamine

and one of five antihistamines:

Brompheniramine	Chlorpheniramine
Dexbrompheniramine	Triprolidine
	Clemastine

Commonly used OTC products that contain one of these decongestants and *one* of these antihistamines are listed in table 14-4.

With these lists in hand, you should be able to step up to the cold and nose counter and make a more informed selection. If you remain confused concerning a selection, ask your pharmacist or doctor for help.

TABLE 14-4
Commonly Used Sustained-Release
OTC Antihistamine-Decongestant
Tablets/Capsules*

Product Name	Active Agent
Actifed 12-Hour Capsules	5mg triprolidine (A)
	120mg pseudoephedrine (D)
Allerest 12 Hour Caplets	12mg chlorpheniramine (A)
	75mg phenylpropanolamine (D)
Chlor-Trimeton Decongestant	12mg chlorpheniramine (A)
Repetabs	120mg pseudoephedrine (D)
Contac Maximum Strength	12mg chlorpheniramine (A
12 Hour Caplets	75mg phenylpropanolamine (D)
Dallergy-D Capsules	12mg chlorpheniramine (A)
	120mg pseudoephedrine (D)
Dehist Capsules	8mg chlorpheniramine (A)
	75mg phenylpropanolamine (D)
Demazin Tablets	4mg chlorpheniramine (A)
	25mg phenylpropanolamine (A)
Dimetapp Extendtabs	12mg brompheniramine (A)
	75mg phenylpropanolamine (D)
Disophrol Chrontabs	6mg dexbrompheniramine (A)
	120mg pseudoephedrine (D)
Drixoral Sustained Action	6mg dexbrompheniramine (A)
Tablets	120mg pseudoephedrine (D)
Isoclor Timesules	8mg chlorpheniramine (A)
	120mg pseudoephedrine (D)
Sinutab Allergy Formula	6mg dexbrompheniramine (A)
Sustained Action Tablets	120mg pseudoephedrine (D)
Travist D	1.34mg clemastine (A)
	75mg phenylpropanolamine (D)
Triamenic-12 Hour Capsules	12mg chlorpheniramine (A)
	75mg phenylpropanolamine (D)
12 Hour Cold Capsules	4mg chlorpheniramine (A)
	75mg phenylpropanolamine(D)

(A) Antihistamine, (D) Decongestant

QUESTIONS AND ANSWERS

1. I'm seventy-one years old and in good health. I don't take any medications. Can I take the full dose of antihistamine decongestant combination medications?

You might be able to, but I'd suggest you begin with the lower doses. Age decreases our ability to metabolize these medications and remove them from our bodies. That means that drugs could accumulate more in a senior citizen than in someone in their late twenties, and that means that you are more likely to experience a side effect. Also, as we age, we become more sensitive to the effects of medications that can cause stimulation (the decongestants and some antihistamines) and drowsiness (the antihistamines). Regardless of your age, never take unnecessary chances with medications.

2. I didn't think that decongestant nasal sprays were good for you, but you recommended them. Why?

Decongestant nasal sprays can be effective and safe medications—as long as you use them as cautioned. The primary concern with these sprays is in the length of time they are used. As said earlier, three to five days should be the rule. If you still need a decongestant after this period of time, use an oral medication.

3. I notice that some of the products in my drugstore's nose and cold section are also good for fever and headache. Will they also relieve nasal symptoms?

If you need to treat nasal congestion, take a decongestant. If you need to treat runny nose, sneezing, and itching, take an antihistamine. If you need to treat both, take an antihistamine decongestant combination medication. If you need to treat pain (headache) or fever, take a separate medication, you will be able to better treat both headache and fever by so doing.

4. Do menthol-containing products offer added relief.

They just smell and feel good to some people.

5. When should I use a rapid-release product, like a liquid or a low-dose tablet?

Infants and young children need liquids for two reasons: liquids taste palatable and the dose can be adjusted to meet their needs. You can't adjust the dose of most tablets to accommodate infants and most young children. Also, older adults and some younger adults find that they cannot take the larger doses (because of side effects) in sustained-release products, but can use liquids and low-dose tablets.

CHAPTER 15

TAKING SOMETHING EXTRA FOR YOUR RUNNY NOSE: IPRATROPIUM BROMIDE SPRAY

RUNNY NOSE is the end result of the outpouring of secretions from thousands of mucus-producing glands in the lining of the nose. These glands discharge their mucus when signaled to do so by the nervous system. Although antihistamines do provide relief for many people with rhinitis, sometimes nothing antihistamines, decongestants, corticosteroid sprays, or cromolyn sprays seems to work. This is probably because none of these medications interfere sufficiently with the signals from the nervous system to the mucus-secreting glands.

IPRATROPIUM BROMIDE TO THE RESCUE
Ipratropium bromide is a medication with the unique ability to block signals from the nervous system to mucus-producing glands. It is not an antihistamine, decongestant, corticosteroid (chapter 16), or cromolyn (chapter 17) product, and it can be most effective for the treatment of runny nose.

Ipratropium bromide is so new that at the time of this writing the drug is not available for nasal use in the United States. Studies in England support its usefulness in the treatment of runny nose, and its use in rhinitis is currently being studied in the United States. It is available here under the name Atrovent as a metered dose inhaler for use in asthma and bronchitis. When it becomes available for treating runny noses, its brand name will be Atrovent Nasal Spray. In order to understand how Atrovent works, let's take a look at how runny noses happen.

Reflexes, Nerve Signals, And Runny Noses

Reflexes and nerve signals have everything to do with runny noses. A reflex is an involuntary response to a stimulus. It begins in an organ, like the nose. It then travels through the nervous system to the brain or spinal column and is then transmitted back to the organ through other nerve pathways to cause a response. A classic example of this is accidentally touching something hot. The stimulus, heat, sets in motion a process that begins with a signal that travels via nerve fibers to the brain, which interprets this as pain and quickly signals the arm to remove the hand. The entire reflex reaction occurs within milliseconds. The reflexes in your nose that control your production of nasal mucus can be described as having three components:

1. **The Stimulus:** For runny noses this stimulus can come in the form of a variety of agents, including chemicals released during allergic or other inflammatory reactions as well as irritating particles and chemicals.

2. **The From-To-From transmission of Nerve Signals:** The signal must travel *from* your nose to your brain or spinal cord, then back *from* the brain or spinal cord to your nose. All of this takes place within very tiny nerve fibers faster than the blink of an eye.

3. **The Response:** On returning to the nose, the signal is passed to nasal mucus-producing glands, mucus is released, and the result is a runny nose. Ipratropium bromide blocks the signal so that it cannot be communicated to the nasal mucus-producing glands. No signal, no mucus. No mucus, no runny nose.

To understand how ipratropium bromide blocks this signal,

recall the discussion of receptors in chapter 3. The mucous glands in your nose have receptors as well. In this case, these are receptors for the chemical agent acetylcholine, which transmits the signal from the nerves to the mucous glands. In order for acetylcholine to cause mucous glands to release their fluids, it must attach to a receptor on a mucous gland. When ipratropium bromide attaches to the receptors in your nose, acetylcholine cannot link with them and, thus, cannot transmit the signal. Hence, no mucus production; no runny nose.

Four Advantages OF Ipratropium Bromide

1. It greatly reduces runny nose.
2. It is used as a spray. Therefore, you receive very small doses, and those doses are applied directly onto the tissue where it will work.
3. Because it is used in such small doses, generalized side effects rarely, if ever, occur.
4. It does not cause sedation or stimulation, as do the antihistamines and decongestants.

Ipratropium Bromide (Atrovent) Nasal Spray: Use And Effects

When it becomes available for nasal problems, Atrovent will be a nasal spray, and the typical recommended dose will be two sprays in each side of your nose either 2 or 3 times daily It will first come as a 0.03 percent solution, later as a 0.06 percent solution. Completed and published studies suggest that the more concentrated solution (0.06 percent) may be more effective in treating runny noses caused by the common cold.

Indications for Ipralropium Bromide. So far ipratropium bromide has been shown to be effective in reducing or relieving the runny nose component of several common nasal disorders:
The common cold
Perennial allergic rhinitis

Nonallergic perennial rhinitis
Temperature (cold/hot) induced rhinitis
Gustatory rhinitis (chapter 8)

When first released, it is likely that Atrovent Nasal Spray will be recommended for the control of runny nose. The studies that have been completed and published show that Atrovent Nasal Spray 0.03 percent is both safe and effective in patients with the forms of rhinitis listed above. When first released, it is likely to be used after other medications have been tried and have failed rather than as a first-line treatment for runny nose. However, my guess is that once it is discovered by physicians in general, and the public, this will change, and that ipratropium will become a first-line medication for runny noses.

Contraindications of Ipratropium Bromide. Ipratropium bromide is contraindicated only in people who are allergic to it. This is a very, very rare occurrence.

Side Effects of Ipratropium Bromide. Side effects are confined to the nose and mouth. As you might expect, since it reduces nasal mucus and is sprayed into the nose, the most common side effect is dry nose. The next most common side effect is dry mouth. This also makes sense, since after it is sprayed into the nose it is swallowed. Infrequent other side effects include nasal irritation, nasal crusting, dry mouth, and nasal bleeding seen in some patients on high doses. Each of these side effects is usually not severe enough to cause discontinuation of the medication and can be diminished by reducing the number of sprays per dose.

It is important to note here that ipratropium bromide will not affect your sense of smell, cause the mucociliary clearance mechanism in your nose to malfunction, lose its effect on the control of runny nose with prolonged use, cause changes in the cells of the lining of your nose, cause rebound nasal stuffiness, or affect your blood pressure, heart, or vision.

Do Not Take Ipralropium Bromide If You Have Any of the
Following Medical Conditions:
    Narrow-angle glaucoma
    Urinary retention
    Pregnancy
    Nursing mothers

What Will Come In The Future For
Ipratropium Bromide?

My guess is that, after the first product is released, there
will be another release of a stronger product. After that I would
not be surprised to see this compound and either a nasal decongestant spray or a nasal corticosteroid spray combined. However, neither of these will be available for several years to come.

Drug Interaction With Atrovent Nasal Spray

There are no studies or reports indicating any adverse reactions as a result of using ipratropium bromide with other medications. It is safe to use with antihistamines, decongestants,
nasal steroid sprays and cromolyn sodium nasal spray.

QUESTIONS AND ANSWERS
1. Will this spray cause nasal congestion as do the OTC
nasal decongestant sprays?
The problem you are referring to is called rebound or chemical rhinitis and was discussed in chapters 9 and 12. This has
not been reported to occur with ipratropium bromide.

2. Does it help nasal congestion?
It helps runny nose better than any other symptom. However, in some people, it helps nasal stuffiness as well. Just how
it does this is not completely understood.

CHAPTER 16

TAKING ANTI-INFLAMMATORY MEDICATIONS: THE CORTICOSTEROID NASAL SPRAYS

SOME AGENTS CAN REVERSE or even prevent the development of chronic inflammation of the lining of your nose, a condition present in many forms of rhinitis and responsible for persisting uncomfortable nasal symptoms and a generally twitchy nose. Hence, their classification as anti-inflamatory medications.

There are two types of nasal sprays that reduce inflammation of the lining of the nose in chronic rhinitis: the corticosteroid nasal sprays and cromolyn sodium nasal spray. This chapter is about the corticosteroid nasal sprays. Cromolyn sodium nasal spray is the topic of chapter 17.

THE CORTICOSTEROIDS

Corticosteroids are substances produced naturally by your adrenal glands. They regulate a broad range of bodily activities and are marvelous antiinflammatories.

All of the corticosteroid-type medications share a common molecular structure. Hence, they act similarly in the body.

193

However, each agent is produced by changing that common structure just a little, and that change is enough to give it properties different from each of the other corticosteroids.

Side Effects Of Oral Or Injected Use

You may have heard or read that corticosteroids produce terrible side effects. All of the corticosteroid type medications— if taken by mouth or by injection and on a regular basis—can produce very serious generalized side effects (table 16-1). These do not occur with the use of the new nasal corticosteroid sprays discussed below, when used at recommended doses.

TABLE 16-1
Side Effects Associated with the Prolonged
Use of Oral or Injectable Corticosteroid-Type Drugs

Side Effects Associated with Brief Use
Appetite increase
Indigestion
Mood changes: depression, irritability, psychosis

Side Effects Associated with Use for Long Periods of Time
Cataract formation
Easy bruisability
Increases blood pressure
Loss of blood supply to the hip joint
Osteoporosis
Puffiness of the face, back, and abdomen
   secondary to increased fat deposits
Streaking of the skin
Thinning of the skin
Ulcers: stomach, duodenal
Wasting of muscles, especially arms and legs

The First Corticosteroid Nasal Spray

Decadron Turbinaire was the first corticosteroid nasal spray developed and was introduced in the United States in the 1960s.

Its generic name is dexamethasone. Physicians hoped that it would be the answer to their prayers: that it would work well in the nose and have no significant general body effects. Dexamethasone worked wonderfully in the nose, but even when used only as a nasal spray, it was absorbed and acted on the body in general as strongly as if the same dose had been taken by mouth. Because of its ability to act on the body in general, dexamethasone cannot be used as a nasal spray on a regular (daily or near daily) basis for long periods of time without the possibility of developing severe, generalized side effects. However, it remains a very effective agent when used for a brief period of time, and it is superb in helping break the addiction to OTC nasal decongestant sprays.

The newer corticosteroid nasal sprays—bearing trade names of Beconase, Vancenase, and Nasalide—come close to every rhinitis sufferer's dream: they work well in the nose and rarely cause any significant systemic effects when used within the recommended dose ranges. As a result, these medications can be used daily for extended periods of time. Let's examine these new remedies in more detail.

The Corticosteroid Nasal Spray

Beconase/Vancenase. Generic name: beclomethasone diproprionate. Beconase and Vancenase are, in fact, the exact same product sold by two different companies under different common names. Allen & Hanburys manufactures the Beconase line and Schering Corporation manufactures the Vancenase line.

Beclomethasone was first introduced into the United States in the 1970s. Then, it was available only as a metered dose inhaler, similar to an asthma inhaler, but designed to spray medication into the nose. Since then, it also has been introduced as a water-based spray solution, and the delivery apparatus of both of the metered inhalers (Beconase Nasal Inhaler/Vancenase Pockethaler) have been redesigned to improve delivery of the medication into the nose. Each actuation of any of the spray solutions or metered inhalers delivers 42 micrograms of beclomethasone diproprionate into the nose. The usual dosage for Vancenase AQ and Beconase AQ is 1 or 2 inhalations in each nostril two times a day. The usual dosage for Vancenase Pockethaler and Beconase Nasal Inhaler is one inhalation in each nostril three times a day.

Nasalide. Generic name: flunisolide. This product was first introduced into the United States in the mid 1970s as a nasal spray. It is not available as a metered dose inhaler. The spray device is calibrated so that each squirt delivers 25 micrograms of flunisolide into the nose.

Most adults require two sprays in each side of the nose 2 to 3 times a day to obtain control. Once control has been obtained, the dose can be reduced to the minimum that will continue to provide control.

Nasacort. Generic name: triamcinolone. It is available as a metered dose inhaler and is calibrated so that each spray delivers 55 micrograms of triamcinolone into the nose. The beginning dose can range from two puffs each side of the nose each AM to two puffs each side of the nose twice daily. The higher dose may work more rapidly Like all nasal corticosteroid sprays, optimal relief may take as long as three weeks. Once relief has been obtained the dose should be gradually reduced to the lowest that continues to provide relief. If relief has not been obtained after three weeks of use, discuss this with your doctor.

How The New Corticosteroids Nasal Sprays Work

Chronic rhinitis usually refers to chronic inflammation of the lining membrane of the nose. This results in a frequent runny, weepy, stuffy, itchy nose usually accompanied by postnasal drainage and sneezing. In addition, the inflammation creates a state of increased responsiveness, or twitchiness. This means that the nose is more easily triggered by a host of allergic and/ or nonallergic agents.

Nasal corticosteroid sprays can deter all of these symptoms and reduce the likelihood of inflammation recurring, as long as the spray is used regularly. Exactly how these agents work is not completely understood. However, what is known is that (1) they block the formation and release of histamine and other inflammation-causing chemicals from cells, (2) they reduce the number and type of inflammatory cells present in the nasal mucosa, and (3) they decrease the sensitivity of the nerves that cause sneezing. These actions go a long way toward reducing inflammation and controlling nasal symptoms.

While nasal corticosteroids are very effective in relieving nasal congestion, runny nose, sneezing, and itching of the nose, they are less effective in relieving postnasal drip and not at all effective in alleviating eye symptoms. They can, however, help improve your ability to smell. When you have an impaired sense of smell as a result of chronic rhinitis, it is because what little air does flow through your nose does not pass across the olfactory (sense of smell) area high in your nose. Nasal corticosteroids can help your sense of smell by reducing the swelling of the membrane lining your nose, thus allowing more air to flow through your nose and, specifically, more air to flow high into your nose and across the area of smell, where it is sensed by the olfactory apparatus.

Generally speaking, here is what you can expect from using these sprays:

1. Gradual improvement—not the immediate-but-temporary relief you might get from using OTC nasal decongestant sprays. Be patient. Maximum benefit from nasal corticosteroid sprays may take from one to three weeks to become apparent.
2. Regular use. In order for these sprays to work, they must be used regularly every day.
3. Twice to three times a day dosing. Most require at least twice daily use for beneficial effects.
4. Good relief of nasal congestion, runny nose, sneez-

ing, and itching, less effective relief from postnasal drip, and no relief from eye symptoms.

5. If you have nasal polyps, your response time to these drugs may be much longer than 10 days.

6. If you have not gotten significant relief after three to four weeks of regular, twice-daily use, you should notify your physician. He or she may want to reevaluate your nasal problem and/or treatment program.

7. Once improvement occurs, reduce the dose gradually to the smallest dose required to control your symptoms.

8. Around 60 to 90 percent of people who use nasal corticosteroid sprays attain complete control of their symptoms.

Reasons Why You Might Not Respond To Nasal Corticosteroids

Although most rhinitis sufferers do respond to nasal corticosteroids, these medications do not work well for everyone. The explanations include the following:

- Failure to use the medication regularly or frequently enough.
- Discharging the medication into the nose improperly toward the nasal septum—rather than toward the back of the nose, in the natural direction of air flow.
- Not ensuring that your nose is open before using: Blow your nose to clear it of obstructing mucus. Use a nasal decongestant spray if necessary to ensure proper flow of air through the nose.
- Nasal polyps.
- An anatomical abnormality (such as a deviated nasal septum).
- Other medications you are taking (such as for control of blood pressure).

If you have not gotten a good response after faithfully using a corticosteroid nasal spray for three to four weeks, check with your doctor.

Uses For Nasal Corticosteroid Sprays

Nasal conditions in which nasal corticosteroid sprays are indicated include the following:
- Seasonal allergic rhinitis
- Perennial allergic rhinitis
- Nonallergic rhinitis (vasomotor)
- Nasal polyps (prevent recurrence of polyps following surgical removal)
- Chemical rhinitis (the nose-drop or nose spray nose)

Recommended Dose/Frequency Of Administration

Table 16-2 outlines the recommended dose and frequency of administration of the currently available nasal corticosteroid sprays.

Contraindications For Corticosteroid Nasal Spray

There are two general contraindications to the use of corticosteroid nasal sprays:

1. An allergic or hypersensitivity reaction to either the corticosteroid or one of the additives in the spray you plan to use, manifested by sneezing, congestion, generalized itching, coughing, wheezing, fainting, etc.
2. An untreated but significant infection of the lining membrane of the nose.

NOTE: If you are having pain in your nose and/or blowing copious amounts of pus, perhaps with blood intermixed, from your nose, talk to your doctor before you use one of these sprays.

Side Effects Of Corticosteroid Nasal Sprays

The side effects of corticosteroid nasal sprays are generally mild and limited to the nose. Systemic side effects are possible at higher-than-recommended doses.

TABLE 16-2
Recommended Dose/Frequency of Administration of the
Currently Available Nasal Corticosteroid

Product	Dose per Puff/Spray
Decadron Turbinaire	*Adults:* 2 sprays each side of nose 2-3 times daily *Children: (6-12 yrs):* 1-2 sprays each side of nose 2 times daily
Beconase AQ Spray/Vancenase AQ Spray	*Adults and Children > 6 yrs:* 1 or 2 inhalations 2 times daily *Children < 6 yrs:* not recommended
Beconase Nasal Inhaler/Vancenase Pockethaler	*Adults and Children > 12 yrs:* 1 inhalation each side of nose 2-4 times daily *Children 6-12 yrs:* 1 inhalation 3 times daily Children <6 yrs: not recommended
Nasacort Nasal Inhaler	*Adults and children 12 yrs and older:* 1 to 2 puffs each side of nose once daily
Nasalide Spray	*Adults:* 2 sprays each side of nose 2 time daily *Children 6 to 12 yrs:* 1 to 2 sprays each side of nose 2 times daily to 2 sprays each side of nose 3 times daily *Children < 6 yrs:* not recommended

Common side effects include burning, stinging, and irritation of the lining of the nose.

Less common side effects include aggravation of bronchial asthma (by accidentally inhaling the solution into the lungs during spraying), headache, light headedness, nausea, nose bleeding, and rebound nasal congestion (if your nasal congestion worsens with use rather than improves). Rare but possible side effects include a decrease in function of the adrenal glands, allergy to the product or an additive, glaucoma (alert doctor if you have a family history of glaucoma), injury of the nasal septum (the wall that divides the nose into right/left sides), sore throat, thrush, and watering of the eyes.

Special Cautions For The Use Of Corticosteroids Nasal Sprays

The first caution is really a point of common sense: if these sprays are used when your nose is significantly congested, they will not pass far enough into your nose to help. Therefore, before using, be sure your nose is open before spraying them in. If necessary, use nasal decongestant sprays before using the nasal corticosteroid sprays for the first few days of corticosteroid spray use.

Next, the nozzle of the spray should never be pointed toward your nasal septum when you spray your nose. This can injure your septum, as discussed above. It should be directed straight back into your nose, following the direction of air flow through the nose.

If you develop thrush (a yeast infection in the mouth and throat), while using nasal corticosteroid sprays, stop using the spray and treat the thrush. The likelihood of your developing this can be reduced if you simply gargle with water after using the spray or metered inhaler.

If you are using nasal corticosteroid sprays while you have a bacterial infection of your nose, ears, or sinuses, be sure that you also take an antibiotic.

If your nose begins to burn, bleed or generally becomes irritated while using these sprays, stop using them and discuss your symptoms with your doctor.

Last, *never* exceed the recommended dose. If the prescribed dosage does not provide relief, consult your doctor.

QUESTIONS AND ANSWERS

1. Are the corticosteroids used in these sprays the same as the corticosteroids I've been reading about that the wrestlers, football players, and other athletes use?

No, they aren't. Those steroids are a completely different type of medication. In truth, those steroids are actually male hormones.

2. I heard you can get a hole in your nose from these things. Is that true?

If you misuse corticosteroid sprays you can cause an injury to your nasal septum (the bone that divides the nose into two sides) that can result in a hole in the septum. I have seen this on only two occasions and both patients were positioning the nozzle of their steroid spray so that it was discharging directly into the nasal septum, rather than into the nasal passageway. As discussed above, these sprays should be discharged in the direction of natural air flow.

3. My grandmother took corticosteroids for her asthma and she got osteoporosis (softening of the bones) and swelling (fat buildup and fluid retention) of the face and upper body. Will that happen if I take nasal corticosteroids?

One reason why nasal corticosteroids were developed was to have a "steroid" product that would not cause the same general side effects as corticosteroid products taken by mouth. Generally speaking, you should not develop any significant general side effects from the use of nasal corticosteroids as long as you adhere to the manufacturer's recommended dose and frequency of administration.

4. You've warned us about getting hooked on nasal sprays, but now you say that nasal sprays are great medications. I'm confused.

The sprays I have warned you about getting "hooked" on are the OTC nasal decongestant sprays, not the corticosteroid sprays. In fact, if you get hooked on the decongestant sprays, one of the agents your doctor will prescribe to help break your addiction are the corticosteroid nasal sprays.

5. *I have an ulcer, so my doctor says that I can't take corticosteroids. Would nasal corticosteroid sprays fall into this category?*
No. Your doctor is referring to steroid shots and pills. I am unaware of any patient whose ulcers were worsened by the use of nasal steroid sprays. Nasal corticosteroid sprays are not absorbed into your system sufficiently to exert an adverse effect on your ulcers.

CHAPTER 17

TAKING PROPHYLACTIC MEDICATION: CROMOLYN SODIUM NASAL SPRAY

Cromolyn sodium, manufactured by Fisons Corporation and available in the United States as Nasalcrom Nasal Solution since the early 1970s, was the first allergy prophylactic medication developed and marketed worldwide. A prophylactic medication is defined as one that acts as a preventative against disease. Cromolyn sodium functions as a prophylactic medication because it prevents the allergic process from developing. No process, no symptoms. This is in contrast to the other medications for allergic rhinitis-antihistamines, decongestants, corticosteroids, and ipratropium bromide—which act to relieve the symptoms caused by the allergic process, but do not alter the process itself.

THE BASICS OF CROMOLYN SODIUM

How Cromolyn Sodium Works
SINCE THE EARLY '70s, much has been learned about this remarkable medication. Its list of actions currently includes the following:

- Preventing the release of mediators from mast cells
- Preventing the accumulation of inflammatory cells in the lining of the nose
- Blocking both early and late allergic reactions
- Inhibiting the action of cells that cause inflammation

As discussed earlier, it is the chemical mediators released during allergic reactions that cause the persistent inflammation characteristic of chronic rhinitis. Because of its ability to prevent the release of these chemicals into the nasal tissue, cromolyn sodium is widely prescribed by physicians as an allergy "blocking" drug. Of note is that cromolyn sodium is not an antihistamine, a decongestant, or a steroid.

Cromolyn Sodium: Nasalcrom Nasal Solution

Nasalcrom Nasal Solution is the only form in which cromolyn sodium is available for use in the nose, and it is distributed only by prescription. It is formulated to deliver 5.2 milligrams of cromolyn sodium per spray and comes in 13 milliliter and 26 milliliter bottles. The smaller bottle delivers about 100 sprays; the larger delivers approximately 200 sprays. In general, the larger bottle is a better buy in terms of cost per spray.

The recommended dose is as follows: Adults and children older than six years can take one spray in each side of the nose 3 to 4 times a day. If needed, the dose may be increased to 6 times a day. However, many physicians recommend a larger beginning dose: two sprays on each side of the nose 4 times a day.

Like most products that are unique, cromolyn sodium is expensive. You would do well to shop around for the best price before getting your prescription filled. There is only one Nasalcrom Nasal Solution, and no generic equivalent, so quality will not suffer in your attempt to get the best price.

CROMOLYN SODIUM, YOUR NOSE, AND THE REST OF YOUR BODY

Which Nasal Symptoms Respond Best To Cromolyn Sodium?

The nasal symptoms best helped by cromolyn sodium are watery, runny nose and sneezing. Nasal congestion and post-nasal drainage do not respond as well.

Indications for Cromolyn Sodium

The manufacturer's package insert accompanying a bottle of Nasalcrom lists only one indication: "allergic rhinitis." Clinical experience shows that its use should be considered in the following conditions:

- Seasonal allergic rhinitis
- Perennial allergic rhinitis
- Occupational allergic rhinitis
- Possibly effective in most forms of nonallergic, nonanatomic rhinitis

It has not been shown to be helpful in treating either vasomotor rhinitis or chemical rhinitis.

What To Expect When Using Cromolyn Sodium

If you have seasonal allergic rhinitis, you should expect a significant reduction or even clearing of your symptoms during your allergy season. Here are some tips for the effective use of Nasalcrom Nasal Solution:

• For best results, cromolyn sodium should be begun two weeks before the pollen season begins, used regularly throughout the season, and not discontinued until the pollen is no longer in the air.

• If you have perennial allergic rhinitis, you should expect a gradual reduction in your symptoms with *regular* use.

• If you have some other form of rhinitis in which the actions of cromolyn sodium might warrant your giving it a try, look for gradual improvement with prolonged use.

• If, like some of my patients, you have an isolated problem, such as an allergy to your brother-in-law's cat and you experience a flare-up of your nasal symptoms every time you go to his home, you may find that two sprays of cromolyn sodium on each side of the nose about 15 minutes before going into his home, followed by two more sprays on each side of the nose every four hours while there, will offer protection. This doesn't always work, but it works often enough that it's worth a try. If you have an allergy to an agent at work to which you are exposed only occasionally, cromolyn sodium could be used in a similar manner to prevent symptoms.

Side Effects Of Cromolyn Sodium
Sneezing is the most common side effect of cromolyn sodium. This is followed by burning and stinging, bad taste in the mouth, nasal bleeding, and increased postnasal drip. A rash is the least common side effect.

Contraindications For Cromolyn Sodium
The only contraindication to the use of this medication is if you are allergic to it, which is very rare—so rare, in fact, that in over 20 years of practical experience, I have *never* had a patient develop an allergy to cromolyn sodium.

Warnings Regarding Cromolyn Sodium Nasal Solution
Like so many products, the safety and efficacy of cromolyn sodium nasal solution has not been established regarding use during pregnancy, lactation, and in children younger than six years.

QUESTIONS AND ANSWERS

1. When do I need to consider using cromolyn sodium?
The first line of defense in treating most forms of rhinitis are the antihistamines and/or decongestants. If these agents taken as directed do not provide the relief you need, then consider using cromolyn sodium nasal spray.

2. I understand that cromolyn sodium will also help asthma. How does it help the lungs when I spray it into my nose?
Cromolyn sodium does help asthma, but not in its nasal spray form. Cromolyn sodium is available in two other forms for use with asthma: (1) a metered dose inhaler (a "puffer"), which is discharged into the mouth and inhaled into the lungs, and (2) as a solution for use in a breathing machine:

3. I used cromolyn sodium nasal spray, but my nose remained congested. Why?
Cromolyn sodium is not a nasal decongestant, so nasal congestion is not helped much by sodium cromolyn. It is most effective when your most troublesome symptoms are watery, runny nose and sneezing.

4. My cousin has used cromolyn sodium nasal spray for more than two years. Is this safe?
Yes, it is. Many people who use this product must do so several times a day every day. Its intended use is for prevention, or prophylaxis of symptoms. That requires, for many, regular, daily use.

5. Are there any medications I should not take while I am taking cromolyn sodium?
Unlike the antihistamines and decongestants, there are no medications that are known to interact adversely with cromolyn sodium nasal spray.

CHAPTER 18

THE PROS AND CONS OF ALLERGY SHOTS

ALLERGY SHOTS, desensitization, hyposensitization, and immunotherapy are different terms for the same thing. Immunotherapy is the term allergists use when referring to allergy shots. Immunotherapy is the process by which a series of injections of gradually increasing doses of extracts of airborne allergens is taken. Only the allergens to which you are allergic are used in immunotherapy. These may include dust mites, mold spores, and grass, tree, or ragweed pollens. Each injection received is just a little stronger than the preceding one until you reach the highest dose that will be given. This dose is frequently called the maintenance dose, because it is the dose that will be repeated, weekly or every other week, throughout your course of immunotherapy. Ordinarily, it will take about three months of regularly administered injections to reach your maintenance dose. This maintenance dose is then continued at regular intervals until you have obtained your maximum relief. An immunotherapy program for airborne allergens generally requires a minimum of three years of injections.

Immunotherapy works by producing very specific immune

changes in your body. Allergic conditions responding to immunotherapy include the following:
- Seasonal Allergic Rhinitis
- Perennial Allergic Rhinitis
- Insect Sting Allergy
- Allergic Asthma

The focus of this chapter will be on immunotherapy as given for seasonal allergic rhinitis and perennial allergic rhinitis. The other form of allergic rhinitis, occupational rhinitis, is best treated by avoidance measures, and the nonallergic types of rhinitis do not respond to immunotherapy because they are not caused by allergens.

Most people with perennial allergic rhinitis have nonallergic triggers of their nasal symptoms as well. For example, you might have PAR and be using nasal decongestant sprays too often as well as suffering nasal congestion whenever you are around cigarette smoke, perfumes, or the smell of cleaning chemicals. Your chronic nasal symptoms are in fact caused by the interaction of three different types of rhinitis: allergen triggered rhinitis (PAR), nose-spray triggered rhinitis (chemical rhinitis) and irritant triggered rhinitis (irritant rhinitis). Immunotherapy will help protect you against the allergens causing your perennial allergic rhinitis. It won't help you break the nose- spray habit or keep cigarette smoke from twitching your nose. Other measures will have to be used to help you break the nose-spray habit and reduce your response to irritating odors.

Before You Take Immunotherapy

Just because you have nose symptoms that act like allergy doesn't mean that you are allergic. The first step in determining whether or not your nasal symptoms would benefit from immunotherapy is to be certain that you have allergic rhinitis. That requires your doctor to ensure that you actually make IgE antibodies (allergic antibodies) to the common airborne allergens and that it is these allergens that are causing your symptoms. To do this your doctor must take a very detailed medical history, perform a physical examination, and then do skin or serological (blood) tests to confirm the presence of IgE antibodies to common airborne allergens. Once these allergy tests are obtained, they are correlated with the history and physical examination findings and a treatment program is planned.

The steps that should be taken prior to your beginning any immunotherapy program are summarized in table 18-1.

TABLE 18-1
Before Beginning Immunotherapy

1. Be sure that your nose problem is allergic and not some other problem that causes similar symptoms.
2. Be sure that you have IgE antibodies to airborne allergens (pollens, dust mites, animals, etc.).
3. Your symptoms should be uncomfortable and poorly controlled by avoidance measures and medications.
4. Be sure that you are willing to take the time to participate in the treatments.
5. Be sure that the physician giving your immunotherapy is experienced in the diagnosis and treatment of allergic rhinitis.

Anyone who embarks on a course of immunotherapy should make a commitment to complete the entire course of therapy Taking a course of immunotherapy for a few months, stopping it, and then starting it again is a waste of your time and money. If immunotherapy is to be effective, a high dose of allergen extract must be given regularly over a prolonged period of time. If you stop and start on the program, you will never achieve the dose needed, nor will you take it long enough for it to help.

Immunotherapy is time consuming and expensive. If you are going to make such a commitment to time and funds, then for goodness' sake seek out a specialist in allergic diseases. Ask for references from your regular physician or friends who have undergone immunotherapy.

What Is An Allergist?

An allergist is a physician who, on completing medical school, trained at least three years and passed an examination to become a fully qualified specialist in either internal medicine or in pediatrics. After that, he or she must undergo at least two years of highly specialized training in allergy and immunology. Mere completion of this training does not qualify one as a specialist. To be recognized as a specialist in allergy, a physician must next become certified by the American Board of Allergy and Immunology, a conjoint board of the American Board of Internal Medicine and the American Board of Pediatrics. This requires the passing of a comprehensive examination that assesses the doctor's basic knowledge as well as diagnostic and treatment skills with a variety of allergy and immunology problems. All told, specialists in allergy and immunology are required to complete five years of training and pass two difficult specialty examinations before they can be recognized as allergy specialists. Your county/parish medical society should be able to provide you with a list of board-certified specialists in allergy and immunology. If not, you can always call the American Board of Allergy and Immunology, in Philadelphia, at (215) 349-9466, the American College of Allergy and Immunology, in Chicago, at (708) 359-2800, or the American Academy of Allergy and Immunology, in Milwaukee, at (414) 272-6071.

Allergens Used In Immunotherapy For Allergic Rhinitis

Immunotherapy is directed against airborne allergens such as dust, dust mites, elm pollen, mountain cedar pollen, ragweed pollen, rye grass pollen, and mold spores. Your allergy shots should contain the airborne allergen(s) to which you are allergic, and nothing else. Under special circumstances cat extract can be used, but allergy to cats, unless you are a veterinarian or some other individual who *must* otherwise be in contact with a cat, avoidance is the best treatment (chapter 10).

How Immunotherapy Works

The key "immune" players in allergic reactions (see chapter 3) are IgE antibodies, mast cells, basophil cells, and the chemicals released from these cells, called mediators. It is on these antibodies, cells, and mediators (table 18-2) that immunotherapy exerts its effects.

TABLE 18-2
What Immunotherapy Does

Immune Factor	Before Immunotherapy	After Immunotherapy
IgE antibodies	Present Increase during pollen season	Reduced Blunting of seasonal increase
Mast cells	Release mediators	Release is blunted
Basophil cells	Release mediators	Release is blunted
Chemical mediators	Released	Release is blunted
IgE "blocking antibody"	Present	Presence increased Binds allergen so it cannot bind with IgE antibodies

Before immunotherapy, IgE antibodies (the allergy antibodies) increase in number after a season of exposure to the pollen(s) to which you are allergic. After immunotherapy, the level of these antibodies decreases and no longer or only slightly increases after a season of exposure. The general trend is for the IgE antibody level to decrease during your course of immunotherapy. Before immunotherapy, your mast cells and basophil cells bind with the IgE antibodies and release chemicals whenever these antibodies react with something to which you are allergic. After immunotherapy, there is a decreased release of chemical mediators from these cells after exposure to an allergen. Decreased release means fewer symptoms for you.

We all have the ability to make antibodies to anything that invades our body: food, viruses, bacteria, and airborne allergens. We all make a certain amount of IgG antibody to airborne allergens. Immunotherapy causes us to make much more IgG antibody to the allergens in our shots. In theory this antibody functions as a "blocking antibody." Ideally, there should be so much more of IgG than IgE antibody that when an airborne allergen invades your system, it binds with IgG rather than IgE. Since the binding of IgG and allergen does not set off an allergic reaction, fewer chemicals are released into your nasal tissue and you suffer fewer symptoms.

Immunotherapy works through a *combination* of these effects, rather than via a single effect.

What Immunotherapy Does Not Do

Although immunotherapy can be very effective in reducing the frequency and severity of your allergy symptoms, it does not provide a permanent cure for your allergy problems. It also can greatly reduce your need for medication, but it rarely completely eliminates your discomfort. Nor does it make avoidance measures unnecessary. In fact, faithful avoidance may greatly enhance the result you get from immunotherapy. The effects may last for a few years after you've stopped the injections, but it is common for them to recur. If they do recur and become uncomfortable, you can take another course of injections.

Side Effects Of Immunotherapy

There are five possible side effects to an allergy shot:
1. A small area of redness (smaller than the size of a
   quarter), swelling, and itching at the site of injection that

begins within a few minutes of your receiving the injection and that goes away within 1 to 2 hours.

2. A larger reaction (larger than a quarter but smaller than a silver dollar in size), swelling, and itching at the site of injection, beginning a few minutes after the injection and clearing in 1 to 2 hours.

3. A very large area of swelling (inches of swelling), redness, and itching that begins some 4 to 6 hours after a shot, lasts a number of hours, then gradually resolves itself over 24 to 48 hours.

4. A mild generalized reaction that begins within 30 minutes of receiving an injection and consists of generalized itching, hives, and some coughing and mild wheezing.

5. A severe, life-threatening reaction; this typically begins within 20 to 30 minutes after an injection, and takes the form of severe shock.

The very mild reactions are common, large local reactions are less common, very large local reactions even less common, generalized mild reactions are uncommon, and the life threatening reactions are very, very rare. A recent study of deaths from allergy skin testing or allergy immunotherapy shots revealed 46 deaths since 1945. Considering the millions of such injections given each year—some say as many as 10 million each year—such a catastrophe is rare indeed. In fact, the chances of your dying from an allergy injection are 30 times less than those of dying from being struck by lightening, 2,000 times less than dying from the effects of smoking or passively smoking cigarettes, and 16,000 times less than dying in an automobile accident. I mention this because sometimes one hears scare messages about immunotherapy, implying that it carries a high risk of life-threatening reaction. Such messages are in fact, unfounded, providing the physician knows and understands what he or she is doing. Again, you should be absolutely certain that the physician in charge of your immunotherapy is properly trained and experienced in the safe and effective administration of this therapy. Other guidelines for safe immunotherapy are listed in Table 18-3.

How Often To Take The Shots

I'd like to share with you the immunotherapy schedule most often followed in my office. We begin with very dilute extract, containing very little allergen. Injections are initially given twice weekly, each injection containing a little more allergen than the last. This pattern continues for about 12 weeks. At this point, the patient should have reached the highest dose we give. This dose will be continued weekly for four weeks. If there are no large local or more serious reactions up to this point, all subsequent injections throughout your course of injections will be given every 14 days.

TABLE 18-3
Additional Guidelines for Safe Immunotherapy

1. Be sure that the physician providing the treatment is appropriately qualified.
2. If you had a reaction from your last shot, always tell the doctor or his or her nurses about this before you take your next shot.
3. Stay in the doctor's office 30 minutes after your shots.
4. Stay on schedule. You can't reach your maintenance doses if you do not.

Highly Questionable Immunotherapy Procedures

There are a variety of unproven methods of administering immunotherapy being given patients in the United States today. These controversial methods are practiced almost exclusively by physicians who are not specialists in allergy and immunology, a comment that should speak for itself. So, if immunotherapy

has been recommended for you or your child, ask questions:
- Is the physician providing the immunotherapy a specialist in allergy and immunology?
- If not, is there such a specialist in your area?
- Is the physician providing the immunotherapy using a method considered unproven or controversial by most allergy specialists? (Those using such methods are *fully aware* of their unproven or controversial nature.)
- What are the reasons that the physician is recommending an unproven or controversial mode of treatment rather than using a scientifically proven method?
- What are the reasons that you or your child are not being referred to a properly trained specialist for consultation before such is undertaken?

This is no time to be bashful. Immunotherapy is an expensive, time-consuming form of therapy. Ask questions. If you are going to receive a controversial form of therapy, you deserve to know that it is considered controversial. So, get answers. It is only through asking questions and receiving answers that you will be able to make an informed decision regarding the recommended immunotherapy plan.

Unproven methods can be offered for several reasons, none of which are very flattering to the profession of medicine. First, neither the vulnerable public nor most of the nonallergist medical world have any idea which methods are considered proven and which are not. Second, fear of restraint-of-trade lawsuits by physicians who employ unproven methods prevents local, state, and national medical societies that are aware of these problems from acting on their concerns. Third, federal regulations (imposed by the Federal Trade Commission) make it very difficult, if not impossible, for the medical profession to properly control the actions of its members. Unfortunately, it is the patients who suffer from all of this confusion.

Advice: Stick with proven methods of immunotherapy. The names of trained and certified specialists in allergy and immunology in your area can be obtained from the following organizations:

Your local medical society
The American Board of Allergy and Immunology
The American College of Allergy and Immunology
The American Academy of Allergy and Immunology

The Future Of Immunotherapy

The next steps in the improvement of immunotherapy are now being taken. These include the following:
1. Identification of which fractions in each airborne allergen actually cause our symptoms.
2. Modification of these fractions so that, when injected, they produce an even more potent immune response than currently used agents, but cause no significant adverse side effects.
3. Developing standards of quality for all allergens used in immunotherapy.

Not only will these actions improve the effectiveness and safety of immunotherapy, but they will also improve skin tests and blood serum tests for allergy, as these employ the same allergy solutions as does immunotherapy.

QUESTIONS AND ANSWERS

1. I've taken allergy shots for three years for tree pollen allergy. Now, they say that I'm allergic to ragweed pollen and need shots for that. I thought my other shots took care of everything!

Allergy shots are allergen specific. They protect you only to what is in the injection. There is some overlap between certain weeds, some trees, and some grasses, but tree shots don't protect you from weeds, nor do weed shots protect you from grasses, etc.

2. How long does the effect of allergy shots last once I've stopped?

Probably from one to three years. My experience is that the effect lasts closer to three years. You are best protected while taking the shots. This protection will last a varying period of time after you've stopped your shots, but it will not last forever. If you stop shots and symptoms recur, you have the option of taking them again.

3. Can I give my own allergy shots?

There is much discussion among allergists about self injection. Some teach patients how to do this; some absolutely will not. The greatest concern, of course, is the possibility, remote as it may be, of an adverse, life-threatening reaction to an injection while at home, where optimal medical care is not available.

Whether or not patients give themselves shots at home appears to be somewhat dependent upon where they live. In the northeastern United States, it is not a common practice, while in the South it is commonplace.

Although we encourage most patients to come to our office for their shots, some cannot. Many live in rural areas or have work schedules that simply do not permit the frequent office visits required. We teach these people how to give themselves injections. Each is carefully instructed concerning the proper technique of administration, what side effects to expect, what side effects to be concerned about, when to call us, how to stay on the proper schedule, what to do if they miss a shot, and how to use injectable epinephrine should a severe reaction take place. In the 22 years I have been in the practice of allergy, no one in our practice has ever experienced a severe, life-threatening reaction.

The final decision regarding self injections should be based on a thorough discussion of the matter with your physician.

4. If I take immunotherapy will I still have to take allergy medicine?

Since allergy shots reduce your reactivity but do not completely eliminate it, you may have to use medication intermittently or regularly throughout your immunotherapy. You should notice, however, that you require less medication as your program progresses. Some patients rarely require anything other than their shots.

5. *My doctor doesn't believe in allergy shots, but they helped my sister's hay fever. My hay fever is worse than hers. Would shots help me?*

If you want and can benefit from immunotherapy, it should be readily available to you through most allergists.

PART SIX

Complications of Rhinitis

CHAPTER 19

INFECTED SINUSES

THE MEDICAL TERM for what we commonly refer to as our sinuses is the *paranasal sinuses* (*para* means around or near; and *sinus* means space or hollow). The paranasal sinuses are empty spaces in the bones of the face and head that surround and connect with the nasal cavities. They are lined with the same membrane that lines the nose, and drain into the nose cavity via openings called *ostia*. There are four paranasal sinuses:

The Maxillary Sinuses
The Ethmoid Sinuses
The Frontal Sinuses
The Sphenoid Sinuses

Each is named for the bone(s) of the skull in which they lie (figure 191).

What Sinuses Do
As far as we know, the sinuses have six main functions:
1. Lighten the weight of the skull.
2. Act as chambers to resonate our voices.
3. Warm the air as we breathe it.
4. Humidify the air as we breathe it.
5. Protect the interior of the skull from injury.
6. Act as insulators to keep the base of the brain, which is close to the inside of the nose, warm.

to the inside of the nose, warm.

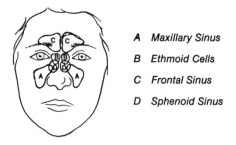

A   Maxillary Sinus

B   Ethmoid Cells

C   Frontal Sinus

D   Sphenoid Sinus

Figure 19-1: **The Paranasal Sinuses**

Sinusitis

Sinusitis is a common complication of chronic rhinitis, whether allergic, chemical, irritant, or infectious. Sinusitis is a medical term that most people use to refer to any infection of the sinuses. Literally, sinusitis means an inflammation of the sinuses. That inflammation can be caused by a variety of factors, but the most common cause of inflammation of the sinuses is infection.

Generally speaking, sinusitis evolves in a four-step sequence.

1. Mucus Production Increases. Whatever the triggering factor—allergen, infectious agent (cold virus or bacteria), chemical pollutant, or toxic agent—the end result is stimulation of the membrane lining of the sinuses to make substantially more mucus than normal.

2. Ciliary Clearance of Sinus Debris Decreases. At the same time that more mucus is being made, the little hair-like cells lining the mucous membrane (the cilia) lose their ability to sweep the mucus out of the sinuses.

3. Closure of the opening of the Sinuses into the Nasal Cavity Occurs. While the cilia are losing their ability to clear the sinuses of debris, chemicals, and germs, the openings of the sinuses into the nasal cavity close because of swelling of the lining of the nose, making clearing impossible.

4. Infectious Agents Flourish. In the now dark, wet environment of the nose, trapped viral or bacterial agents multiply and sinus injury continues.

Infectious Organisms That Commonly Cause Sinusitis

1. **Viruses:** The same organisms that cause the common cold are the most common causes of sinusitis.
2. **Bacteria:** A variety of bacteria cause sinusitis. Names like *Diplococcus, hemophilus influenza* (not the flu germ), beta *Streptococcus* (as in strep throat), *E. coli* (as in diarrhea), and *Staphlococcus aureus* are the most common.

Conditions Causing Increased Susceptability To Sinusitis

A number of other conditions can increase your chances of developing infected sinuses. These are summarized in table 19-1. The three most common predisposing factors are recurring colds, allergy, and being addicted to nose sprays or drops.

Table 19-1
Conditions Predisposing You to Sinusitis

Recurring colds	Tumors
Allergy	Foreign bodies
Nose spray abuse	Swimming
Enlarged adenoids	Diving
Nasal polyps	Flying
Deviated nasal septum	Smoking or passive smoking

HOW ALLERGY CAUSES SINUSITIS

As detailed in chapter 3, allergy reactions go through several stages. The early allergic reaction can cause swelling of the sinus openings by rapidly leaking fluid into the tissue lining the nose and sinuses. The late allergic reaction is an inflammatory reaction and acts in the same way as if a bacteria or virus had inflamed the lining of the nose and sinuses.

The Two Types of Sinusitis

There are two types of sinusitis: acute and chronic. Whether you have one or the other depends upon how long your symptoms have been present.

Acute Sinusitis. If your sinusitis has been present for less than three weeks, it is called *acute*, meaning that it is of short duration. In older children and adults, there are three typical symptoms of acute sinusitis:
1. Pain or a sensation of pressure in the face over the area of the infected sinus is common. This is made worse by bending over, straining, jogging, or going down stairs.
2. A cloudy nasal discharge, from one or both sides, or a cloudy postnasal drip.
3. Fever, which is not a part of chronic sinusitis.

In younger children symptoms are not specific. A nighttime cough that doesn't respond well to cough medications may be the only symptom.

Chronic Sinusitis. This is the term used to describe sinusitis present for longer than three weeks. It is not unusual for this condition to continue for months. In older children and adults there are three typical symptoms:
1. Chronic nasal congestion or stuffiness
2. Frequent, or almost constant colds
3. A persistent cough

In younger children, typical symptoms include the following:
1. The child seems to always "keep a cold"
2. Cough, particularly a nighttime cough, is a nuisance
3. Recurring ear infections

In all age groups, a cloudy postnasal drip, otherwise unexplained bad breath, and recurring ear infections are common associations. Facial pain and fever are not frequent in chronic sinusitis.

A pattern I frequently see in young children, older children, and adults is one of recurring symptoms. In other words, symptoms come, are treated, clear, but recur in one to two weeks. They are again treated and clear, but recur. This repeated occurrence of symptoms should raise the suspicion of chronic sinusitis.

Do You Have Sinusitis Or Rhinitis?

Your rhinitis may have turned into sinusitis if you suffer the symptoms outlined in table 19-2:

TABLE 19-2
Your Rhinitis May Have Become Sinusitis If ...

1. It hurts. There may be pain in your cheeks, at the base of your nose, or around your eyes.
2. You have a fever.
3. You are blowing pus from your nose.
4. Your "cold" won't go away.
5. You have a cough that won't clear.
6. Your cold clears, but recurs, then clears, but recurs, etc.

Diagnosing Sinusitis

If you go to the doctor with the symptoms discussed above, he or she will examine your nose and throat. It is quite possible that during this examination your sinusitis will be identified, as your doctor may spot pus seeping from one or more of the openings of your sinuses into the nasal passageways.

A sinus X-ray may be needed. If you have sinusitis this usually shows either swelling in the lining of your sinuses or pooling of pus in one or more sinuses.

Occasionally, a very sophisticated type of study called a CAT-scan will be needed. This is a much more detailed X-ray of your sinuses and better defines the extent of your sinusitis. CAT-scans are not done on everyone with sinusitis because they are not usually necessary to diagnose and treat the problem, and because they are expensive. However, occasionally the physical examination and regular sinus X-ray results leave either the diagnosis or the full extent of the problem in doubt. Under these circumstances a CAT-scan can be most helpful.

Disorders That Masquerade As Sinusitis

Not everything that looks and feels like sinusitis will be sinusitis. You should be aware of the common conditions that might seem to be sinusitis, but that are not:

1. Angioedema (allergic swelling). This is a localized swelling of the skin and tissues under the skin due to an allergic reaction to something. If it occurs on the face, around the nose or eyes, it could be mistaken for sinusitis.

2. Temporal Arteritis. This is an inflammation of a major artery running across the temple. It usually involves only one side and is usually painful to the touch.

3. Cellulitis. This is an infection of the skin and the tissues under the skin. The skin is usually red, warm to the touch, and painful. If this occurs over the cheeks, at the base of the nose, or around the eyes, it could be mistaken for sinusitis.

4. Headache. Since there is facial pain with acute sinusitis, it is possible that some mild forms of headache, and even migraine, could be mistaken for sinusitis. Most of the time this is not a hard differentiation to make.

5. Neuralgia of the Trigeminal Nerve. This is a condition in which intense pain shoots across the face along the path commonly followed by the trigeminal nerve. Trigeminal refers to the fact that this nerve branches and follows three courses across the face. The pain felt with this is intense, like that caused by placing ice on a cavity of a tooth. This is very different from the usual sinus pain, which is dull and pressure like.

    6. Toothache. Your upper teeth are very close anatomically to the maxillary sinus cavities. In fact, they can actually push up against the sinuses. Should one of these teeth become infected, that infection can irritate the lining of the sinuses and can cause discomfort similar to sinusitis. This is usually easy to tell as tapping of the teeth, chewing, or ingesting hot beverages do not usually bother sinusitis, but will aggravate an inflamed tooth.

    7. Tumors. Many tumors of the nose cavity do not produce symptoms until they have grown enough to invade the surrounding tissue. At this point, it is common for them to produce pain. Since that pain is usually noted around the nose, the first impression is that one has sinusitis. However, the other more typical symptoms of sinusitis are usually absent.

Treatment Of Sinusitis

    There are two general principles in the treatment of sinusitis:

    1. Promote opening of the sinuses. This can be done using the medications listed below:

    • **Topical Decongestants.** Nose sprays or drops can be used, but, as in the treatment of rhinitis, they should never be used more than 3 to 5 days in a row. Since sinusitis will usually require two to four weeks of treatment, I have found that using these agents for five days, stopping use for seven days, using them again for five days, and so on throughout the course of treatment of sinusitis minimizes the development of an "addiction" to nasal sprays or drops.

    • **Oral Decongestants/Antihistamine.** The regular use of decongestants, such as a pseudoephedrine product, is a method commonly employed throughout the treatment course of sinusitis. They provide added decongestion both during and when "off" topical decongestant nasal sprays. If you have allergic rhinitis and it is your allergy season, then the addition of an antihistamine or the use of a combination antihistamine-decongestant product might be in order.

• **Topical Nasal Corticosteroid Sprays.** These are good anti-inflammatory agents and are commonly taken throughout the treatment of sinusitis.

• **Oral or Injectable Corticosteroids.** These agents can hasten the reduction of the inflammation and are frequently taken at the beginning of treatment for sinusitis.

2. *Treat the infection.* Antibiotics are the best defense here. The most common type of antibiotics used to treat sinusitis are:

Amoxicillin
Amoxicillin combined with clavulanate
Trimethoprim-Sulfamethoxazole
Erythromycin plus sulfisoxazole
Cefaclor

Because of the spectrum of bacteria it kills, amoxicillin is a good first-choice antibiotic for the treatment of sinusitis. Against certain organisms amoxicillin with clavulanate, trimethoprim-sulfamethoxazole, erythromycin plus sulfisoxazole, or cefaclor may be more effective. *Penicillin allergic patients*, however, should not take amoxicillin-containing antibiotics because amoxicillin is a penicillin derivative. They also should use cefaclor-type antibiotics with caution, because cefaclor-type antibiotics sometimes cause allergic reactions in penicillin-allergic patients. If you are allergic to penicillin, *always tell your doctor* of this before taking any antibiotic.

If you have sinusitis, in all likelihood, you will take antibiotics for at least 14 days. At the end of that time, if you still are not well, you will be given another two to four weeks of antibiotics. In general, if you have been through two courses of antibiotics such as this (some four to six weeks of treatment) and still are not well, you may require sinus surgery. Remember that if you develop sinusitis it is important to take the medications exactly as directed and for as long as directed even if you begin to feel better before the medication is used up.

Complications Of Sinusitis

Most of us take sinusitis for granted. We assume that it is just an infection and that if we take some medication, all will be well. Fortunately, that is usually the case. However, sinusitis can become seriously complicated. A sinus filled with pus is nothing less than an abscess sitting in one of the bones of the skull, and abscesses, if not drained, can extend to surrounding areas including the eye, the brain, and the adjacent bones. The serious complications of sinusitis include brain abscess, meningitis, infection of the tissue and skin around the eye, infection of the bone surrounding the sinus, the development of chronic bronchial infections, and significant aggravation of bronchial asthma.

QUESTIONS AND ANSWERS

1. I've heard that people with chronic sinusitis shouldn't take aspirin. Is this true?

Only if you have something called Sampter's syndrome, also called aspirin allergy or aspirin idiosyncrasy. Sampter's syndrome was defined in chapter 8 and discussed in terms of the simultaneous occurrence of chronic sinusitis, nasal polyps, bronchial asthma, and an abnormal reaction to aspirin.

2. Is there any particular allergen that tends to cause more sinusitis than any other?

No. Any allergen or combination of allergens can cause changes in your nose sufficient to trigger sinusitis. Cats can do it, birds can do it, mites can do it, pollen can do it, etc.

3. How long does it take to get over sinusitis?

Weeks, sometimes longer, but never less. This is why you undergo treatment for at least two weeks, and frequently for three to four weeks.

4. My son has had a cough for three months. Does he have sinusitis?

Not every child with a persistent cough has sinusitis, but it is a very common cause of chronic cough. There are other causes of chronic cough such as unsuspected asthma, tumors in the chest, and other problems that should be considered if his cough has been going on this long. These can be explored with your child's doctor.

5. My X-rays didn't show sinusitis, but my CAT-scan did. Is there any significance to this discrepancy?

If your symptoms suggested sinusitis and the usual sinus X-rays did not confirm it, your doctor showed good judgment in requesting a CAT-scan of your sinuses. As discussed earlier in this chapter, one advantage of the CAT-scan is that it shows more detail than regular sinus X-rays, hence can sometimes confirm a diagnosis of sinusitis when the regular X-rays could not.

CHAPTER 20

INFECTED EARS AND FLUID
IN THE EARS

TWO OF THE MOST common complications of rhinitis are infected ears (acute otitis media) and fluid in the ears (otitis media with effusion). Although both occur in adults as well as children, these problems are much more common in children.

FACTS ABOUT INFECTED EARS AND FLUID IN THE EARS

1. Some 10 million children are treated each year for otitis.
2. Fifty percent of children have at least one episode in the first 12 months of life.
3. About 75 percent of children have had at least one episode by the time they are two years old.
4. One-third of children will have had three or more bouts of otitis by the time they reach their second birthday.
5. Otitis is a problem mainly for children less than three years of age and remains a common problem for children through the early school years.
6. Fifty percent of children with infected ears will have persisting fluid in their ears for as long as one month after the infection has been treated.
7. These two conditions—infected ears and fluid in the ears—are the most common reasons for surgery (ear tubes) in the United States and Great Britain.

Who Is At Risk For Ear Problems?

Table 20-1 lists the conditions that, if present, predispose you or your child to having either acute otitis media or otitis media with effusion.

TABLE 20-1
Conditions Associated with the Development of
Acute Otitis Media and Otitis Media with Effusion

Infectious rhinitis
Allergic rhinitis
Enlarged adenoids
"Immature" eustachian tube
Nonallergic rhinitis
Nasal polyps
Undertreatment of a previously infected ear
Injuries to the middle ear or Eustachian tube
Tumors, benign or malignant
Congenital abnormalities (cleft palate)
Sudden changes in altitude
Gross obesity
Some forms of paralysis
Low functioning thyroid gland

THE ANATOMY OF YOUR EAR
Figure 20-1 and the description that follows outline the anatomy of the ear pertinent to nose and sinus-related problems.

Three Divisions Of The Ear

The Outer Ear. These are the parts of the ear that are visible from the outside as well as the tube leading to the eardrum.

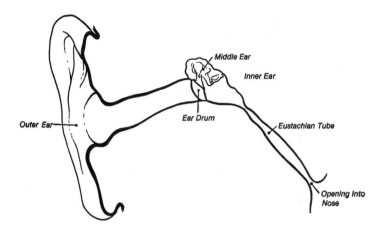

Figure 20-1: The Three Divisions of Your Ear

The Middle Ear. This is a chamber, normally filled with air, that includes the eardrum and the little bones inside the ear through which the eardrum works.

The Inner Ear. This is the system that transfers the motions of the eardrum into signals that are carried to the brain, where they are interpreted as sounds.

The Eustachian Tube

An extension of the middle ear chamber, the Eustachian tube connects the middle ear to the back of the nose. The middle ear and Eustachian tube are both lined with a membrane very similar to that of the nose, with mucus-producing glands and cilia to sweep the mucus and its trapped debris from the middle ear, through the Eustachian tube, and out into the back portion of the nasal cavity. Abnormal Eustachian tube function is the root cause of recurring ear infections and fluid.

How the Eustachian Tube Functions. It may surprise you to know that the Eustachian tube is collapsed, or closed, most of the time. Normally, it opens only briefly during swallowing, yawning, sniffing, and activities associated with straining. When it does open, air passes into and out of the middle ear, fluid is swept (by cilia) from the middle ear into the nose, and then the tube quickly closes again.

The Eustachian tube has three main functions: First, it ventilates the middle ear. Second, it lets air into and out of the middle ear, allowing the middle ear to "breathe." Third, because it is closed most of the time, the Eustachian tube serves as a highly effective barrier, preventing unwanted debris such as germs, irritants, and allergens from entering the middle ear. It also provides the route by which mucus made in the middle ear is expelled into the rear portion of the nasal cavity.

Immature Eustachian Tubes. It is believed that the reason behind the frequency of ear infections in some young children is a delayed maturation of their Eustachian tube. Such a tube does not function normally: it is more collapsible than a normal tube, doesn't ventilate the ears properly, doesn't act as an effective barrier to injurious agents, and doesn't permit the ciliary mechanism to clear the ear normally. Add a cold virus, a bacterial infection of the sinuses and nose, irritants such as cigarette smoke, and airborne allergens to the world of this abnormal tube, and you get ears that either are easily infected or form and trap excessive fluid. Fortunately, as the child matures, so does the Eustachian tube (it grows, gets better support from its surrounding tissue and bone, and attains normal function). This maturation process occurs between ages three to six. Beyond six years of age, middle-ear infections are much less common than earlier in life.

THE PROBLEM OF OTITIS

How Does Rhinitis Cause Otitis?

A basic component of every form of rhinitis is inflammation, the degree of which varies from person to person. When the nose is inflamed, it is common for the Eustachian tube and ear to become involved in that inflammation. When that happens, the Eustachian tube swells, sometimes to the point of complete closure, trapping air behind. When this happens two other important events take place:

1. The air trapped in the middle ear cavity gets absorbed into the blood stream via the rich network of tiny blood vessels surrounding the middle ear. The absorption of this air produces a relative vacuum in the middle ear. This change in pressure within the ear causes fluid to ooze from the walls of blood vessels into the ear cavity. The swelling of the Eustachian tube also blocks the circulation of blood and tissue fluid from the ear and provides another means by which fluid accumulates in the middle ear. If the process stopped here, you would have otitis media with effusion (OME)—i.e., fluid in the ear, but no infection associated with it.

2. If an infection-causing agent such as a virus or a bacteria is trapped in the middle ear cavity, the result will be an infected middle ear, otitis media (OM).

Oitis Media

The term *otitis media* (OM) means inflammation *(-itis)* of the middle *(media)* ear *(otic)* cavity and refers to the fact that the lining of the middle ear cavity and the Eustachian tube have become inflamed. There are two general types of inflammatory reactions in the middle ear:

1. Acute Otitis Media (AOM)
Almost everyone has had this problem once in his or her childhood. First, you got a cold, then an earache and fever, and the pediatrician told you that you had an "ear infection." Whatever virus or bacterial infection was causing your coldlike symptoms had inflamed the lining of the middle ear cavity and Eustachian tube. Your Eustachian tube swelled and closed, fluid from the inflammation (pus) formed in the ear, pushed on the eardrum, and you got one heck of an earache. You actually had developed an abscess in the ear.

Adults with AOM will experience fever, general malaise, reduced hearing in the infected ear, and perhaps dizziness or even ringing in that ear.

Children with AOM will complain of earache and will have fever, but they rarely become dizzy or complain of ringing in the infected ear.

Infants with AOM will have a high fever, be irritable, and pull at or otherwise fidget with their ears.

Treating Acute Otitis Media (AOM). The single most important goal of the treatment of AOM is the elimination of infection from the middle ear cavity Antibiotic medications play the most important role in accomplishing this goal. Amoxicillin (Amoxil, Polymox, Trimox, Wymox) is very often the first antibiotic used, and is commonly taken for 10 to 14 days. However, it should never be used when one is allergic to penicillin. Other antibiotics used to treat AOM include amoxicillin with clavulanate (Augmentin), erythromycin with sulfisoxazole (Pediazole), any erythromycin product (EES, Eryc, Pediamycin, etc.), trimethoprim-sulfamethoxazole (Bactrim, Septra), and cefaclor (Ceclor).

Caution: Up to 15 percent of people allergic to penicillin who take cefaclor-type antibiotics react to those antibiotics. That is because these antibiotics have a chemical structure similar to that of penicillin. If you are allergic to both penicillin and cefaclor-type antibiotics, your doctor will likely treat you with erythromycin, erythromycin with sulfisoxazole, or trimethoprim-sulfamethoxazole.

When AOM complicates chronic rhinitis, decongestants in the form of nasal sprays/drops, or pills, capsules, or liquids by mouth are also commonly used, as discussed in chapter 12.

2. Otitis Media with Effusion (OME)

In this form of otitis, fluid accumulates in the middle ear for the same reasons discussed above, but the ear is not infected by viruses or bacteria. Unlike pus, this fluid can range from being very thin (like water) to very thick (like glue).

If you have an effusion, it is likely that you sense a popping or plugged-up feeling in your ears. You might also notice that you are not hearing as well.

Children with OME, however, may not complain of such ear symptoms. In fact, it might be you or your child's teacher who complains. You might notice that your child doesn't seem to hear you. Your child's teacher might complain about his or her "not paying attention" in class. You both might note a drop in school performance or a change for the worse in behavior. Before you decide that such a change is due to a behavior problem, have your child's ears and hearing tested, as that is the only way to diagnose the ear problem.

Treating Otitis Media with Effusion (OME). There are two goals in the treatment of OME:

1. Removing the fluid from the middle ear cavity. This is first accomplished by encouraging the Eustachian tube to open, thus permitting the middle-ear cavity contents to drain into the nose. Decongestant medications—either nose drops/sprays or medications taken by mouth—can be helpful, as can the corticosteroid nasal sprays (chapter 16).

If the fluid persists for six to eight weeks or more, your doctor may consider the placement of small polyethylene (plastic) devices, referred to as PE tubes, in the eardrum in such a way as to provide an opening between the middle ear and the external ear. This type of surgery usually requires a brief anesthetic, so it is usually done as a day surgery procedure. These devices vary in size and shape, ranging from something that looks like an empty thread spool to a simple tube. A commonly used spool-type device is 2 millimeters in diameter and 3 to 5 millimeters in length.

These tubes allow air to enter the middle ear cavity and equalize the ear and outside air pressures. They also permit fluid to drain from the ear. Both actions help reduce the inflammation of the middle ear lining and Eustachian tube, and that helps reduce swelling and promote the natural drainage of fluid from the ear. PE tubes generally remain in place from 6 to 18 months, working their way out naturally. Yes, you may find one on your child's pillow. These tubes are quite safe, and it is most unusual for them to cause any permanent injury of the eardrum or loss of hearing. Other than hearing better and having fewer infections of the middle ear, most children with these devices never notice they are there.

2. Prevent reaccumulation of fluid in the ear. When possible, the best treatment of any illness lies in prevention. Prevention is accomplished by the proper treatment of the underlying conditions that caused the problem to develop in the first place.

This could be accomplished for OME using a variety of tools depending upon the underlying predominant cause. Avoidance, antihistamine-decongestant medication, nasal corticosteroid sprays, cromolyn sodium, and/or immunotherapy are options for treating the nonanatomic forms of rhinitis.

The anatomic causes of OME and recurring AOM include enlarged adenoids, nasal polyps, tumors, congenital malformations, and other anatomic problems. Generally, the treatment for these anatomic causes is surgical correction.

QUESTIONS AND ANSWERS
1. I thought that if you had recurring ear infections, you should have your tonsils removed. Is this true?

Tonsillectomies used to be common treatment for ear infections, but that is no longer the case. Removing the tonsils does not help recurring ear infections; it is enlarged adenoids that cause the problem. The tonsils are a very important part of our immune system and are producers of antibodies and cells that protect us against infectious illnesses. They should not be removed unless absolutely necessary. The days of having all the children in the family go into the hospital at the same time for removal of the tonsils and adenoids have long passed.

2. My nephew has recurring ear infections and his doctor keeps him on antibiotics continuously during the winter. Can't this prescription prove harmful?
Continuous use of antibiotics is sometimes a necessary step in the management of a child with recurrent ear infections who is just not responding to the more common options. This course of treatment is usually given only during the times of year when upper respiratory infections are common.

3. How can I tell if my child is hard of hearing?
Your child's teacher may complain about his or her not paying attention in class, or there may be a deterioration in his or her schoolwork. If he or she asks you to repeat questions, doesn't seem to know which direction sounds are coming from (turns the wrong way in response to stimulus), keeps the stereo or TV turned up too loud, talks unusually loudly, or is giving you the impression of ignoring you, hearing could be a problem. Speech development in very young children may be slowed if their hearing is diminished.

4. Is it really true that cigarette smoke can aggravate my child's ear problems?
Indeed it is. It also can aggravate his or her nose problem, bronchitis, sinusitis, and asthma. Do your child and yourself a favor: don't smoke.

5. After my son's PE tubes were put in, they fell out and had to be reinserted. Is this normal?
It is not uncommon for PE tubes to come out and have to be replaced. It is not a sign that anything was wrong with them or their placement. It is simply that many tubes are intended to work their way out. Most do so over 6 to 18 months, but some come out sooner. If it happens too soon, they have to be replaced.

CLOSING COMMENTS

YOU'VE LEARNED a lot since chapter 1: how the nose is made, how it works, and the types of symptoms it causes when its normal functions are disturbed. You've learned about allergic noses and problems that masquerade as allergies, and that your nose symptoms may be the result of several different causes acting together or separately

You've learned that where you work can affect your nose and why. You've completed a questionnaire that should help you begin the process of better understanding the types of nasal problem(s) you have, and you have learned about the treatment options available to you:

- Avoidance of dust, mites, mold spores, animal allergens, and foods
- Antihistamines
- Decongestants
- Antihistamine-decongestant combinations
- Nasal corticosteroid sprays
- Cromolyn sodium nasal spray
- Ipratropium bromide nasal solution
- Allergy shots

Finally, you've learned about the most common complications of chronic rhinitis: sinusitis, acute otitis media, and otitis media with effusion.

Being better informed is the first step in obtaining the best care for your nose. Use this book. Refer to it when you have questions. Take it with you to the doctor and discuss your questionnaire with him or her. Take it to the drug store, too, and ask about medications. Your doctor and pharmacist will respect your efforts to be informed and welcome your questions. And your nose will be forever grateful.

APPENDIX I

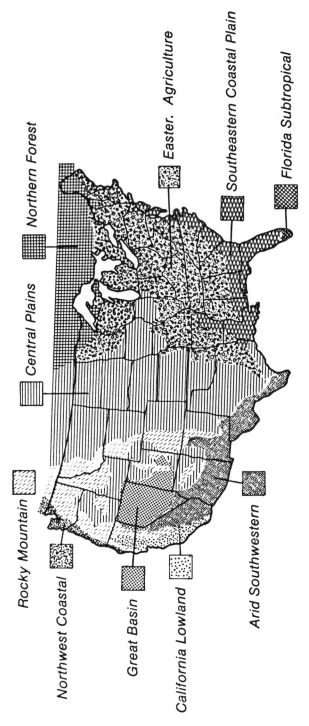

Northern Forest

Easter. Agriculture

Southeastern Coastal Plain

Florida Subtropical

Central Plains

Rocky Mountain

Northwest Coastal

Great Basin

California Lowland

Arid Southwestern

TEN POLLEN REGIONS OF THE UNITED STATES

Region/Pollen	Pollen Season

1. Northern Forest

Tree Pollens	Feb	Mar	Apr	May	Jun	Jul	Aug	Sep	Oct
Alder				▓					
Arborvitae				▓					
Aspens				▓					
Birch				▓					
Fir				▓					
Hazelnut				▓					
Hemlock				▓					
Pine				▓					
Poplar				▓					
Spruce				▓					
Grass Pollens									
Grass					▓	▓			
Weed Pollens									
Ragweed							▓	▓	

2. Eastern Agriculture Forest

Tree Pollens	Feb	Mar	Apr	May	Jun	Jul	Aug	Sep	Oct
Alder		▓	▓						
Ash		▓	▓						
Beech		▓	▓						
Birch		▓	▓						
Box Elder			▓						
Elm		▓	▓						
Hackberry			▓						
Hazelnut	▓	▓							
Hickory			▓	▓					
Maples		▓	▓						
Mulberry			▓	▓					
Oak			▓	▓					
Paper Mulberry		▓	▓						
Poplar		▓	▓						
Sycamore			▓						
Walnut			▓	▓					
Willow			▓	▓	▓				

Region/Pollen	Pollen Season

Weed Pollens	Feb	Mar	Apr	May	Jun	Jul	Aug	Sep	Oct
Hemp						▆	▆		
Kochia						▆	▆		
Marsh elder							▆		
Nettles						▆	▆		
Pigweeds						▆	▆		
Ragweeds							▆	▆	
Russian thistle						▆	▆		
Sagesmugworts						▆	▆	▆	
Sheep sorrel				▆					

3. Southeastern Coastal Plain

Tree Pollens	Jan	Feb	Mar	Apr	May	Jun	Jul	Aug	Sep
Ash			▆	▆					
Birch			▆	▆					
Cedar, red	▆	▆	▆	▆					
Elm		▆	▆						
Hackberry	▆	▆	▆						
Maple			▆	▆					
Mulberry			▆	▆	▆				
Oak				▆					
Pecan			▆						
Poplar			▆	▆					
Sweet Gum			▆	▆					
Sycamore			▆	▆	▆				
Walnut			▆						
Willow			▆	▆					
Grass Pollens									
Burmuda				▆	▆	▆	▆	▆	

4. Florida Subtropical Region

Tree Pollens	Jan	Feb	Mar	Apr	May	Jun	Jul	Aug	Sep
Cypress		▆	▆						
Oak		▆	▆	▆					
Palm			all year						

Region/Pollen	Pollen Season
Grass Pollens	Feb Mar Apr May Jun Jul Aug Sep Oct
Bahia	all year
Burmuda	all year
Johnson	all year
Weed Pollens	
Ragweed	▓░▓░░▓░██░

5. Arid Southwest Region

Tree Pollens	Dec Feb Mar Apr May Jun Jul Aug Sep Oct
Ash	░██░░░░░░░
Cypress	░█░░░░░░░░
Elm	░█░░░░░░░░
Mesquite	░████░░░░░
Mt. Cedar	░█░░░░░░░░
Mulberry	░██░░░░░░░
Olive	░░███░░░░░
Poplar	░██░░░░░░░
Grass Pollens	░░▓░░░░░░░
Burmuda	░░░░████░░
Weed Pollens	
Burroweed	░███░░░░░░
Greaseweed	░░░░████░░
Kochia	░░░░░░████
Rabbit Bush	░░██░░░░░░
Ragweed	░░███████░
Sagebrush	░░██░░░░░░
Shadscale	░░░░███░░░

6. California Lowlands

Tree Pollens	Jan Feb Mar Apr May Jun Jul Aug Sep Oct
Alder	███░░░░░░░
Ash	███░░░░░░░
Birch	░██░░░░░░░
Elm	░██░░░░░░░
Mulberry	███░░░░░░░
Oak	░░██░░░░░░
Poplar	░██░░░░░░░

Region/Pollen	Jan	Feb	Mar	Apr	May	Jun	Jul	Aug	Sep	Oct
Walnut	█	█	█	█						
Grass Pollens										
Burmuda				█	█	█	█	█	█	█
Weed Pollens										
Nettle						█	█	█	█	█
Ragweed							█	█	█	█
Sage								█	█	█
Willow	█	█	█							

7. Northwest Coastal

Tree Pollens

	Jan	Feb	Mar	Apr	May	Jun	Jul	Aug	Sep	Oct
Alder		█	█							
Ash		█	█							
Birch			█							
Box elder		█	█							
Coatal maple				█	█					
Elm			█	█	█					
Hazelnut	█	█								
Oak				█	█					
Poplar-aspen				█	█					
Walnut				█	█					

Grass Pollens

	Feb	Mar	Apr	May	Jun	Jul	Aug	Sep	Oct
Burmuda				█	█				
Blue				█	█				
Orchard				█	█				
Red top				█	█				
Rye				█	█				
Sweet vernal				█	█				
Timothy				█	█				

Weed Pollens

	Feb	Mar	Apr	May	Jun	Jul	Aug	Sep	Oct
Nettle					█	█			
Plantain				█	█	█			
Poverty weed					█	█			
Ragweed							█		
Russian thistle					█	█			
Sagebrush					█	█			
Sheep Sorrel					█	█			

Region/Pollen	Pollen Season

8. Rocky Mountain Region

Tree Pollens	Feb	Mar	Apr	May	Jun	Jul	Aug	Sep	Oct
Alder		■	■						
Ash		■	■						
Birch			■	■					
Elm	■	■							
Oak				■	■				
Poplar			■						
Willow			■	■	■				

Grass Pollens

Similar to Central Plains grasses

Weed Pollens

Low levels above 5000 feet; similar to adjacent areas at lower levels

9. Great Basin

Tree Pollens	Feb	Mar	Apr	May	Jun	Jul	Aug	Sep	Oct
Box elder			■						
Elm		■							
Juniper	■	■	■						
Poplar		■							
Sycamore			■						

Grass Pollens

Generally low levels; species similar to adjacent areas

Weed Pollens	Feb	Mar	Apr	May	Jun	Jul	Aug	Sep	Oct
Greasewood						■	■	■	
Kochia						■	■	■	
Poverty weed							■	■	
Ragweed							■	■	
Russian thistle						■	■		
Sagebrush						■	■	■	

Region/Pollen	Pollen Season

10. Central Plains

Tree Pollens

	Jan	Feb	Mar	Apr	May	Jun	Jul	Aug	Sep	Oct
Ash		▓	▓	▓						
Box elder			▓	▓						
Elm		▓	▓	▓						
Hackberry				▓	▓					
Hickory				▓	▓					
Mt. cedar		▓	▓	▓						
Mulberry				▓						
Oak		▓	▓	▓	▓					
Osage orange					▓					
Poplar			▓	▓						
Sycamore				▓	▓					
Walnut				▓	▓					
Willow			▓	▓						

Grass Pollens

Similar to adjacent regions

Weed Pollens

	Feb	Mar	Apr	May	Jun	Jul	Aug	Sep	Oct
Greasewood					▓	▓	▓		
Hemp					▓	▓	▓		
Kochia					▓	▓	▓		
Marsh elder					▓	▓	▓		
Ragweed							▓	▓	
Russian thistle					▓	▓	▓		
Sagebrush						▓	▓	▓	
Sheep sorrell				▓	▓				
Smotherweed					▓	▓	▓		
Western water hemp					▓	▓	▓	▓	

APPENDIX II

MEDICATIONS REPORTED TO OCCASIONALLY PRODUCE NASAL SYMPTOMS AS A SIDE EFFECT

Medication(s)	TYPE OF NASAL SYMPTOMS PRODUCED				
	Congestion	Run/Drip	Sneeze	Bleed	Dry
Accutane				•	•
Actifed					•
Activase				•	
Adalet	•				
Advil				•	
AeroBid	•		•	•	•
Afrin	•		•		
Aldoclor	•				
Aldomet	•				
Aldoril	•				
Ambenyl	•				•
Ansaid				•	
Apresazide	•				
Apresoline	•				
Apresoline-Esidrix	•				
Azdone		•			
Beconase		•	•	•	
Beconase AQ		•	•	•	
Benadryl					•
Bentyl	•				
BuSpar	•			•	
Calderol		•			

	TYPE OF NASAL SYMPTOMS PRODUCED				
Medication(s)	*Congestion*	*Run/Drip*	*Sneeze*	*Bleed*	*Dry*
Cardizem	•			•	
Cardizem SR	•			•	
Cartrol	•				
Catapres					•
Catapres-TTS					•
Cipro				•	
Clinoril				•	
Colyte		•			
Combipres					•
Comhist LA					•
Compazine	•				
Corgard	•				
Coricidin Spray			•		
Corzide	•				
Cyclomydril Drops					•
Cytotec				•	
Danocrine	•				
DDAVP nasal spray	•				
Decadron Turbinaire				•	•
Deconamine					•
Demi-Regroton	•				
Demser	•				
Demulen		•			
Desyrel	•				
Diapid spray	•	•			
Dibenzyline	•				
Dimetane DC Cough Syrup					•
Dimetane DX Cough Syrup					•
Disopyramide					•
Diupres	•			•	
Diutensen-R	•				
Dramamine					•
Dristan Spray LL		•	•		
Dristan Spray R		•	•		
Elixophyllin Kl Elixir			•		
Emcyt		•			
Enduronyl	•				
Enovid		•			
Esimil	•				
Etrafon	•				

Medication(s)	TYPE OF NASAL SYMPTOMS PRODUCED				
	Congestion	*Run/Drip*	*Sneeze*	*Bleed*	*Dry*
Feldene				•	
Flagyl	•				
4-Way Spray R, M, LL		•	•		
GoLYTELY		•			
Harmonyl	•				
Hismanal				•	
Histaspan D				•	
Hydromox	•				
Hydropres	•			•	
Hytrin	•			•	
Indocin				•	
Intal	•			•	
Intron A	•			•	
Iopidine					•
Ismelin	•				
Klonopin			•		
Limbitrol	•				
Lioresal	•				
Lortab ASA			•		
Loxitane	•				
Lozol			•		
Ludiomil	•				
Marax					•
Matulane				•	
Mellaril	•				
Methergine	•				
Methotrexate				•	
Midamor	•				
Minipress	•			•	
Minizide	•			•	
Mithracin				•	
Moduretic	•				
Motrin				•	
Mykrox				•	
Nasalcrom Spray	•		•	•	
Nasalide Spray	•		•	•	
Navane	•				
Nicorette			•		
Norethin		•			
Normozide		•			

| Medication(s) | TYPE OF NASAL SYMPTOMS PRODUCED | | | | |
	Congestion	Run/Drip	Sneeze	Bleed	Dry
Norpace					•
Norzine					•?
Optimine	•				•
Oreticyl	•				
Ornade Spansule	•				•
Orudis				•	
PBZ Tabs/Elixir					•
PBZ SR					•
Paradione				•	
Parlodel	•				
Periactin	•				•
Permax				•	
Permitil	•				
Polaramine	•				•
Prinivil	•				
Prinzide	•				
Procardia	•				
Prolixin	•				
Protostat	•				
Proventil Inhaler				•	
Proventil Aerosol Solns	•				
Prozac	•			•	
Quadrinal			•		
Raudixin	•			•	
Rauzide	•			•	
Recombivax HB			•		
Regitine	•				
Regroton	•				
Renese-R	•				
Retrovir caps				•	
Robaxin	•				
Rocaltrol		•			
Rogaine solution		•			
Rufen				•	
Ru-Tuss II					•
Salutensin	•			•	
Salutensin-Demi	•			•	
Sectral		•			
Seldane				•	•
Ser-Ap-Es	•			•	

Medication(s)	TYPE OF NASAL SYMPTOMS PRODUCED				
	Congestion	*Run/Drip*	*Sneeze*	*Bleed*	*Dry*
Serpasil	•			•	
Serpasil-Apresoline	•			•	
Serpasil-Esidrix	•			•	
Soma		•			
Stelazine	•				
Tacaryl	•				
Tavist Syrup/Tabs	•				•
Tavist D	•				•
Tegison		•		•	•
Tenex		•			
Tessalon perles	•				
Thorazine	•				
Timoptic	•				
Tolectin				•	
Torecan					•
Trandate		•			
Trental	•			•	
Trexan	•	•	•	•	
Triaminic Exp DH	•				•
Triaminic Drops	•				•
Triaminic TR Tabs	•				•
Tridione				•	
Trilafon	•				
Unasyn				•	
Vancenase		•	•	•	
Vancenase AQ		•	•	•	
Vaseretic		•			
Vasotec		•			
Ventolin Aerosol Soln	•				
Ventolin Syrup				•	
Voltaren				•	
Wellbutrin				•	
Wytensin	•				
Xanax	•				
Yohimex		•			
Zestoretic	•	•			
Zestril	•				
Zorprin		•			
Zyloprim				•	

APPENDIX III

PRODUCT INFORMATION

ALLERGY CONTROL PRODUCTS
96 Danbury Road
Ridgefield, CT 06877
(800) 422-DUST

A complete line of ready-made and custom-made encasements for pillows, mattresses, and springs, filter masks, and allergy control solution.

ALLERGY SUPPLY COMPANY
PO. Box 419
Fairfax Station, VA 22039
(703)323-1111

ALLER/GUARD INC.
Fleming Place Office Parkway
11121 South West Gate Boulevard
Topeka, KS 66604
(913)272-4486

Fisons Corporation
Acarosan Product Manager
755 Jefferson Road
Rochester, NY 14623

Manufacturer of Acarosan powder for house mite elimination, and the Acarex test for the determination of the level of house mites in your house dust.

APPENDIX IV

MANUFACTURERS OF
HOME AIR-FILTRATION UNITS

HEPA (High Efficiency
Particulate Accumulator)
Filters

Airguard Industries
P.O. Box 32578
Louisville, KY 40232
(502) 969-2304

Aluminum Filter Company
1000 Cindy Lane
Carpinteria, CA 93013
(805)684-7651

American Air Filter Company
P.O. Box 37220
Louisville, KY 40233
(502)454-9235

Cambridge Filter Corporation
PO. Box 4906
Syracuse, NY 13221
(315)457-1000

Farr Company
PO. Box 92187
Los Angeles, CA 90009
(213)772-5221

Electrostatic Filters
Honeywell, Inc.
Honeywell Plaza
Minneapolis, MN 55408
(612)870-2142

Trion, Inc.
101 McNeill Road
Stanford, NC 27331
(919)775-2201

Universal Air Precipitator Inc.
303 North Street
New Castle, PA 16103
(412)372-0706

**Filters Using both HEPA and
Activated Charcoal**
Control Resource Systems, Inc.
670 Mariner Drive
Michigan City, IN 46360
(219)872-5519

APPENDIX V

ADDITIONAL READINGS AND SOURCES OF INFORMATION

MEDICAL TEXTBOOKS
Allergic Diseases: Diagnosis and Management
Roy Patterson, M.D.
J. B. Lippincott Company
Philadelphia and Toronto

Allergic Diseases from Infancy to Adulthood
C. Warren Bierman, M.D., and David S. Pearlman,m.a
W B. Saunders Company
Harcourt Brace Jovanovich, Inc.
Philadelphia

Allergy: Principles and Practice
Elliot Middleton, Jr., M.D., Charles E. Reed, M.D., Elliot
F Ellis, M.D., N. Franklin Adkinson, Jr., M.D., John W.
Yunginger, M.D.
The C. V Mosby Company
St. Louis

Physicians' Desk Reference
1991 Edition
Medical Economics Company
Oradell, NJ 07649

GENERAL READING
The Allergy Encyclopedia
The Asthma and Allergy Foundation of America
Penguin USA
120 Woodbine Street
Bergenfield, NJ 07621

The Complete Drug Reference
United States Pharmacopeial Convention, Inc.
Consumer Reports Books
51 East 42 Street
New York, NY 10017

NEWSLETTERS
Asthma and Allergy Advocate
The American Academy of Allergy and Immunology
61 1 East Wells Street
Milwaukee, WI 53202

Rodale's Allergy Relief
Rodale Press
33 East Minor Street
Emmaus, PA 18049

ORGANIZATIONS
American College of Allergy and Immunology
PO. Box 4323
Arlington Heights, IL 60006
(708)359-2800

American Academy of Allergy and Immunology
61 1 East Wells Street
Milwaukee, WI 53202
(414)272-6071

The American Board of Allergy and Immunology
3624 Market Street
Philadelphia, PA
(215)349-9466

Asthma and Allergy Foundation of America
1717 Massachusetts Avenue, N. W
Washington, DC 20036
(202) 265-0265

National Institute of Allergy and Infectious Diseases
National Institutes of Health
Building 31
9000 Rockville Pike
Rockville, MD 20892
(301)496-5717

National Jewish Center for Immunology and Respiratory Medicine
1400 Jackson Street
Denver, CO 80206
(303)388-4461

Index